MW00892931

The Six Pillars of Sports Recovery

*A comprehensive guide on how to recover faster
and outperform at the highest levels*

By
Dr. Rick Rosa

Copyright © 2013 Dr. Rick Rosa
All rights reserved.
ISBN: 1483987442
ISBN 13: 9781483987446

Table of Contents

About the Author:

RICK ROSA, D.C. IS A SPORTS RECOVERY SPECIALIST. Dr. Rosa is the founder of the Six Pillars of Recovery process, which maximizes the recovery process for athletes, thus enhancing their performance.

The Six Pillars of Recovery includes all aspects of recovery such as a scientific approach to recovery, training regimens, supplements, basic nutrition, clothing, psychological testing, and sports-equipment recommendations.

A member of the American Chiropractic Association Sports Council, Dr. Rosa received his doctorate from New York Chiropractic College in 1996 and was hired as a teacher at the college thereafter. In 1996, he began practicing in a multidisciplinary setting, allowing him to experience various approaches to health care and treat all sorts of acute injury and pain syndromes. He is still a member of the postgraduate faculty at New York Chiropractic College and has lectured extensively on many topics and presently teaches other doctors about recovery in sports.

Dr. Rosa has many advanced certifications, including:

- Diplomate in pain management from the American Academy of Pain Management (DAAPM)

- Certified chiropractic sports physician (CCSP) from the American Chiropractic Board of Sports Physicians

- Corrective exercise specialist (CES) from the National Academy of Sports and Medicine

- Performance enhancement specialist (PES) from the National Academy of Sports and Medicine

- Certified Kinesio taping practitioner (CKTP)

He uses many active and passive soft tissue techniques and is certified in the Graston Technique. In addition, due to his extensive work in pro cycling, Dr. Rosa has trained at the famed Serotta International Cycling Institute under Paraic McGlynn in the use of Dartfish motion analysis for bike fits.

Dr. Rosa is pioneering research in the use of Dartfish, a definition video motion-analysis system to evaluate athletes from a movement assessment perspective to find and correct various muscle and joint injuries. He is also trained in the use of musculoskeletal ultrasound that he utilizes in his Virginia locations.

Dr. Rosa considers himself a "professional student" and continually learns more about the latest treatments and techniques to give his patients the best care available.

Dr. Rosa's focus on recovery stems from his clinical background and his ever-present passion for his patients to recover quicker and stronger, both physically and mentally.

His mission has been to provide holistic and complete cutting-edge healing technology with customized treatment programs and a state-of-the-art monitoring service to help athletes recover quicker and stronger, enabling them to perform at their optimum level.

He runs many clinics in the DC metro area, serving athletes and teams.

He provides consulting and training sessions, and he works personally with professional boxers, athletes, and other sports enthusiasts to provide them with the highest level of recovery from heavy sports training.

About the Book:

THE BOOK IS BASED ON THE TALKS AND lectures delivered by Dr. Rosa; it covers the six pillars of recovery; it include all aspects of awareness of state, rest, play, nutrition, physical, and psychology. This book also explains the cutting-edge therapies and technologies employed in sports medicine.

This book is meant for athletes, coaches, trainers, and sports doctors. If you want to know more about physical recovery, better performance, sports supplements, and the latest breakthroughs in sports medicine, then this is the book to read!

Whether you're a trainer, a trainee recovering from an injury, or you're simply in between training, this book can help you boost your performance.

Disclaimer:

THE INFORMATION IN THIS BOOK SHOULD NOT BE considered medical advice. The information in this book is not meant to treat, diagnose, prescribe, or cure any ailment. Always check with your physician before taking any products or following any advice. Always consult your doctor before you start, stop, or change anything that has been previously advised.

This manual is meant for informational purposes only. The author and business owner shall not be held liable or responsible for any loss, damage, injury, or ailment caused or alleged to be caused, directly or indirectly, by the information or lack of information, or use or misuse, of the methods or techniques described in this manual.

Introduction:

HELLO, I'M DR. RICK ROSA; OVER THE LAST few years, I've focused my energy on helping athletes recover faster, perform better, and develop a promising, injury-free sports career for themselves. The passion and drive these athletes possess toward sports is immense, and helping them reach their goals has added, and continues to add, great satisfaction, pleasure, and meaning to my life.

The athlete is the *star*, and the core of an athlete's star quality depends a great deal on physical fitness and athletic energy.

There's nothing more inspiring than watching athletes perform at their peak state. Peak performance inspires everybody and sparks delightful enthusiasm in the watcher; it motivates people to put their lives on hold and come watch a match or cheer fanatically at a sports event.

It's easy to feel the vibrancy and energy of an athlete who is in a peak state—on the other hand, there is nothing more disheartening than watching an aspiring athlete being held back and pinned down by his or her injuries.

We are lucky that we have the tools and technology today to help athletes perform at their highest potential and give them the winning edge.

I believe that with the right kind of training and recovery, any athlete can outshine, outrun, and outperform his or her competition!

In this book I'm going to share with you all the knowledge that I've accumulated over the past few years; in this book we are going to take a holistic approach toward recovery; I'm also going to share with you information about the best supplements, testing devices, and perfor-mance-enhancement strategies. So let's get started.

The Philosophy:

Training and performance take up a major part of an athlete's daily life and schedule. Even though science continues to break through existing limitations and brings innovation to the table, the attitude and knowledge of the average sports-person does not go very deep; such people certainly seldom understand the importance of recovery.

Recovery is just as important as training, yet it seems not many athletes, trainers, or coaches really focus on the aspects of recovery. If the medical and coaching staff intensified the monitoring and augmentation of recovery as the second part of training, the athletes would recover much faster and train harder.

Every day in my clinical practice, we are constantly looking at improving the recovery of patients, not only in an effort to speed up the process, but also to help prevent exacerbation and reinjury.

So then here's the big question: Why not look at the workout as a traumatic event and do everything we can to promote healing? To do so would ensure proper recovery and also improve the speed of recovery.

Over the last twenty years, the role of the sports chiropractor has expanded and increased significantly. From my treating the many local weekend warriors to professional and Olympic-level athletes, I felt that everyone who is involved in sport has the potential to learn important information to be able to act as their own recovery specialists.

There is a reason some athletes get injured all the time, while others have very few injuries during their careers. Part of it has to do with the fact that sports training and recovery is not a purely physical process; it doesn't start and end with the training routine; it stretches a lot beyond the training room. When you take a closer look, it's easy to realize that sports athletes face a lot of mental pressure: they don't get enough rest, some of them are on autopilot mode (low on awareness), and some of them don't pay enough attention to their nutrition.

When you study all these aspects that govern sports performance, it's easy to realize the necessity for creating a comprehensive training and recovery program for athletes that not only covers the physical recovery aspect but also covers the athletes' mental well-being, relaxation, and nutrition strategies. When all these elements blend together, they create the perfect environment for the athlete to snatch the all-important winning edge.

As I studied and researched the elements that govern peak performance, I realized that athletic performance can be improved tremendously if we started focusing more of our energy on recovery. Why not combine cutting-edge healing technology and state-of-the-art monitoring and create customized treatment programs to help athletes recover quicker and stronger, enabling them to perform at their optimum level? After researching, implementing, and testing many different ideas, I began to develop the concept of six separate pillars of recovery. Using these six pillars, I have established recovery plans for athletes that encompass all aspects of healing and recovery.

The Basic Premise of the Six Pillars:

THE SIX-PILLARS PHILOSOPHY BRINGS TOGETHER ALL THE ASPECTS of recovery and provides a well-rounded, holistic approach to help the athlete recover faster and train harder. This comprehensive approach enables a more complete healing process; it prevents further injuries and also speeds up recovery between workouts. Athletes have shown excellent response to the six-pillars philosophy.

The true testing grounds on my theories on recovery were during the 2007 Paris Brest Paris, a ride that has been done in France for over one hundred years, covering over 760 miles, with the riders stopping only for food and a few hours' sleep. In 2007, it was cold and rainy, one person died, and one thousand people dropped out. As a cyclist and runner, I have been able to apply my knowledge to help athletes recover better and faster.

The bottom line is simply this: the quicker you recover, the harder you can apply yourself in the workouts to follow, which leads to greater gains!

It is possible to map out and monitor specific plans for complete recovery.

Sports trainers, athletes, and experts are ideally situated for this role as recovery specialists who can monitor an athlete or team's recovery program and will certainly offer something that is presently not available to most teams. In addition, athletes will become more aware of their recovery state and when indeed they have fully recovered. That being said, athletes can put much more into their workouts, which will ultimately improve their performance.

After reading this book, you will have the basic tools to understand the many aspects of recovery and how to implement them into your practice.

Outline of the Six Pillars:

As mentioned earlier, the six pillars are all about unifying the various disciplines of psychology, physiology, and science to create a comprehensive recovery plan for athletes, so they can recover faster, train harder, and outperform others at the highest level of competition.

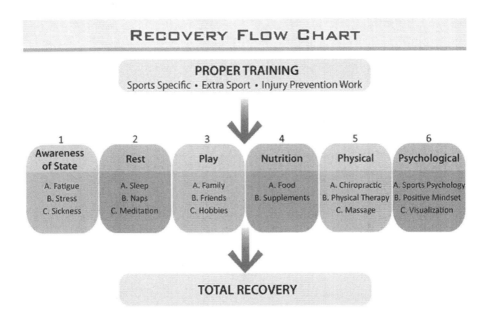

Here's a brief outline of the six pillars of recovery:

1. **Awareness of state**: Using the awareness techniques described in this book, athletes will have the ability to measure how much they have recovered from a workout or sickness. Awareness of state consists of three parts: fatigue, stress, and illness.

<u>Fatigue:</u>

a. Muscle fatigue

b. Neurological fatigue: PNS and CNS

c. Psychological fatigue

d. Environmental fatigue

<u>Stress:</u>

a. Signs of stress

b. Good stress

c. Bad stress

d. Stress pathology

e. Stress and inflammation

f. Stress cancer

g. Oxidative stress

<u>Sickness/Illness:</u>

a. Various pathogens

b. Signs of impending Illness

c. Transmission/ Transmission control

d. Training with illness

2. **Rest:** It is no secret that sleep helps our bodies to heal, recover, and regenerate. Adding naps and meditation can take rest one step further. The following topics need to

be considered to understand the athlete's requirement for rest.

    a. Sleep—stages of sleep

    b. Neurotransmitters and hormones of sleep

    c. How travel affects sleep

    d. Jet lag

    e. Sleep inertia

    f. Sleep aids

    g. Sleep tools

    h. Meditation

3. **Play**: A structured training and recovery plan can be stressful. Maintaining focus indefinitely is impossible, so we need to remember to add stress relievers such as family, friends, and laughter into our lives. The section below titled "The third pillar of recovery: Play" will consider the following:

    a. Importance of family and friends

    b. Hobbies

    c. Laughter

4. **Nutrition:** Food and its impact on athlete performance is no secret; the amount of information in this area continues to grow every day. In addition, supplements can also help the athlete recover faster by reducing inflammation and free-radical formation. The section below titled, "The

fourth pillar of recovery: Nutrition" will consider the following:

   a. Anti-inflammatory diet

   b. Eating clean—avoiding processed food and additives

   c. Supplements

   d. Power foods

   e. Nutrient timing

   f. Hydration

   g. Oxidative stress

5. **Physical:** Adding chiropractic, massage, and physical therapy can make a huge difference when it comes to injury prevention and recovery. Moreover, maintaining proper biomechanics, muscle symmetry, and balance are essential. The section below titled "The fifth pillar of recovery: Physical" will consider the following:

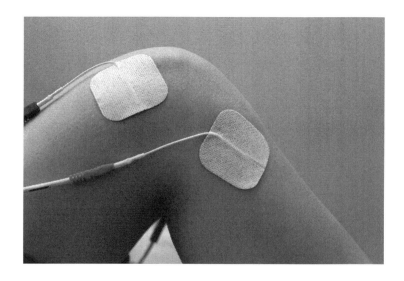

    a. Chiropractic

    b. Physical therapy and recovery modalities

    c. Physical medicine and surgery

    d. Testing methods and recovery monitoring

6. **Psychological:** Methods to balance psychology will be considered in the book's final section.

    a. Psychological skills training: Arousal regulation

    b. Overtraining/Burnout/Injury psychology

    c. Progressive relaxation

    d. Breath control

    e. Biofeedback

    f. Relaxation response

    g. Autogenic training

    h. Cognitive-affective stress management training

    i. Stress inoculation training

    j. Imagery

The First Pillar of Recovery

Awareness

The First Pillar of Recovery: Awareness

What is awareness?

AWARENESS IS THE ABILITY TO FEEL, PERCEIVE, AND to be conscious of the physical and mental state that we are in.

When we are in a state of complete awareness, we are able to sense our state of well-being and react to any condition or event appropriately.

The most common states that we observe in athletes are either a state of partial awareness or a state of complete lack of awareness, which is commonly described as acting in the autopilot mode. This happens mostly because athletes have a lot of concerns and thoughts over how things are going to turn out during the competition; the intense pressure to perform often shifts their awareness from their physical state of well-being to high-pressure, goal-oriented thoughts.

While having a goal-oriented outlook is beneficial, it will work to the athlete's advantage only when the body is completely fit. The body is under constant stress; goal-oriented hyper-drive may actually push the athlete to stretch to extreme limits and thereby lead to burnout. In this state athletes are very likely to ignore the sensations and signals given off by their bodies.

Awareness is a primitive function controlled by the brain stem. The brain stem assesses the sensations in the body and thereby regulates the actions and recovery process of the human being, but, as described earlier, when an athlete faces constant pressure, the cortex (thinking part of the brain) suppresses the function of the brain stem, thereby causing the athlete to completely ignore the sensations in the body.

Since awareness is a function controlled by the brain stem, it is not enough for the athlete to understand the concepts of awareness at an intellectual level; instead the athlete needs to cultivate the ability to feel sensations physically and learn adequate skills to slow down, disengage, step back, and recover completely before engaging in another round of intense training.

Our role as sports physicians is to educate athletes about body awareness and teach them the importance of observing signs and signals from their bodies. This will allow them to recognize signs of physical exhaustion at a very early stage.

Let's have a look at the three major areas that can affect the performance of an athlete. These are the three major areas where an athlete needs to have high levels of awareness.

These areas are

1. Fatigue,

2. Stress, and

3. Sickness.

Fatigue:

What is fatigue?

The words that athletes use to describe fatigue are *tiredness, lethargy, exhaustion, sleepiness,* and *weariness*. Fatigue has many possible causes; it often manifests as an inability to continue functioning at the athlete's normal ability.

How is muscle fatigue different from clinical fatigue?

Clinical fatigue and muscle fatigue are different in their basic characteristics. Clinical fatigue is described as the motor deficit, perception, or decline in mental function accompanied by a gradual decrease in the force capacity of muscles (Bailey et al. 2007; Friedman et al. 2007; Hacker and Ferrans 2007).

However, muscle fatigue represents a transient decrease in the capacity to perform physical actions. There is no global definition for muscle fatigue. Different physiology experts have varied opinions regarding the definition of muscle fatigue. Let's look at some of the well-known definitions of muscle fatigue:

- "Intensive activity of muscles causes a decline in performance, known as fatigue." [1]

- "Performing a motor task for long periods of time induces motor fatigue, which is generally defined as a decline in a person's ability to exert force." [2]

- "CNS administration of caffeine increased treadmill run time to fatigue." [3]

- "A fatiguing task was performed with the muscles of the left hand until the muscles were exhausted." [4]

- "Fatigue is known to be reflected in the EMG signal as an increase of its amplitude and a decrease of its characteristic spectral frequencies." [5]

- "The sensation of fatigue is the conscious awareness of changes in subconscious homeostatic control systems." [6]

According to these definitions, muscle fatigue can be a motor deficit, a perception, or a decline in mental function, or it can signify a decline in the force capacity of muscle or a reduction in muscle force, a change in electromyographic activity, or an exhaustion of contractile function.

However, to avoid debate, experts in sports medicine look at muscle fatigue as an exercise-induced reduction in the ability of muscle to produce force or power, whether or not the task can be sustained. [7]

It is important to understand the distinction between muscle fatigue and the ability to continue the task. Task failure is not a measure of muscle fatigue; instead, any reduction in the maximum force or power that the involved muscles can produce is considered muscle fatigue; it can develop quickly after the onset of sustained physical activity.

An athlete is said to experience muscle fatigue when suffering from reduction in maximum force or power that can be exerted by the muscles.

How can muscle fatigue be measured?

Muscle fatigue can be measured as a reduction in muscle force, change in EMG activity, or exhaustion of contractile function. By comparing tetanic stimulation and maximal voluntary contraction force, one may reveal whether fatigue is of central origin, or whether peripheral mechanisms are involved. [8]

Does gender influence fatigue?

Yes. Researchers have identified many gender-specific differences in muscular fatigability. These factors include

- Muscle mass,

- Substrate utilization, and

- Neuromuscular activation. [9]

Female athletes tend to produce lower absolute muscle forces when compared to males while performing the same relative muscular work. This leads to a lower rate of oxygen demand in females during exercise. [10] These factors improve the oxygen delivery and metabolic by-product (primarily carbon dioxide) removal during submaximal exercise and lead to delayed onset of fatigue in females. This phenomenon is described as the female fatigue resistance advantage in submaximal sporting and exercise events.

Research has also shown that males show a greater glycolyctic capacity, whereas females display greater capacities for fat oxidation (fat breakdown). [10] Studies have shown that that males tend to become more fatigued than females in both maximal and submaximal exercise. [10] Further electromyography (EMG) activity confirms the proportionately lower following fatiguing muscular contraction in males compared to females.

How can trainers utilize this knowledge?

Since females are less prone to get fatigued than males in submaximal workload, the trainer may choose to give the female client a greater volume of workouts at the same submaximal intensity with more sets and repetitions; this will help the female client attain maximum benefits.

Since males have a higher tendency to fatigue during submaximal workouts, they may benefit from additional recovery time, both between sets and between days of training, in order to recover completely. On the other hand, females may be able to perform at high intensity with less rest between sets and a smaller recovery period between training sessions.

What causes muscle fatigue?

In simple terms, the cause of muscle fatigue can be a malfunction of one or several of the physiological processes that enable the contractile proteins to generate a force necessary to carry out the activity. However, in reality, there can be more than one cause for muscle fatigue. Muscle fatigue can be caused by many different factors ranging from accumulation of metabolites within the muscle fibers to the generation of an inadequate motor command in the motor cortex. [11]

So then how do can we break it all down to understand its components?

Other forms of fatigue:

For the purpose of simplicity, fatigue can be divided into the following categories:

1) Metabolic fatigue

2) Neurological fatigue

     A. peripheral nervous system

     B. central nervous system

3) Psychological/emotional fatigue

4) Environmental/travel fatigue

1. Metabolic fatigue:

Metabolic fatigue is a term usually used to describe a reduction in contractile force due to the direct or indirect effects of the reduction of substrates or accumulation of metabolites within the muscle fiber. This may be caused due to a simple lack of energy to fuel contraction, or due to an interference with the ability of Ca^{2+} to stimulate actin and myosin to contract.

When does metabolic fatigue occur?

Metabolic fatigue usually occurs as a result of demanding training sessions that last longer than one hour or due to multiple sessions in one day or over the course of many days.

Metabolic fatigue can also be cumulative if there are inadequate nutritional and hydration strategies.

What causes metabolic fatigue?

As discussed earlier, metabolic fatigue is usually seen in prolonged exercises. Examples of these sports include cycling, cross-country skiing, and distance running.

The most important prerequisite for proper athletic function is efficient muscle contraction. Muscle contraction depends on ATP, which is generated through certain metabolic pathways. The primary supplier of ATP is mitochondrial respiration (aerobic metabolism in the mitochondrion of the cell).

The two most important components for mitochondrial respiration with regard to fatigue are blood glucose and muscle glycogen. Reduced levels of blood glucose and muscle glycogen have been associated with the onset of fatigue in sustained exercise events. [12] Even though fats (triglycerides) are readily available for ATP production, they usually take more time to be broken down.

Another important factor that causes metabolic fatigue is dehydration. Dehydration can be noticed in endurance sports such as hiking, cross-training events, and long-distance running. The body temperature and cardiovascular function are often affected in cases of fluid loss and insufficient fluid intake and replacement.

There is also a constant release of bodily heat due to repeated muscle contraction during these sustained events; this can lead to high body temperatures and cause hyperthermia. According to sports research (Fitts 1994), rising body-core temperatures can lead to fatigue in both the contracting muscles and central nervous system.

Due to improper fluid balance, athletes may experience fluid loss, which in turn reduces the blood flow to contracting muscles; since the muscles require high blood flow, the heart tends to overwork to compensate for the shortage in blood flow; this increases the heart rate and stresses the cardiovascular system. This can lead to metabolic fatigue.

Signs of metabolic fatigue:
The athlete fatigues sooner than normal or struggles to finish an event.

2. Neurological fatigue:
Neurological fatigue can be due to central nervous-system causes or due to peripheral nervous-system fatigue.

Peripheral nervous system fatigue:
This may be seen during periods of short, high-intensity workouts; strength training; plyometrics; and sports bouts.

Motor nerves stimulate muscle fibers (which exist in groups of hundreds). The muscle fibers, along with the motor nerve that stimulates them, are known as a motor unit.

During periods of high-intensity workouts, the neurotransmitters (chemical messengers) become impaired and are unable to carry the nerve's excitation message to the muscle via the neuromuscular junction.

This mechanism results in a decreased efficiency of the muscle fibers' ability to contract (Gardiner 2001).

In addition, low intensity, steady-state workouts can also cause fatigue. PNS fatigue is noted as a reduction in localized force production and can occur without evidence of metabolic fatigue.

Central nervous system fatigue:

This type of fatigue can be related to low blood glucose levels when the athlete is injured, is pushed into the sport, or is psychologically stale: without drive and motivation.

This type of fatigue can occur with or without metabolic, PNS, or environmental fatigue.

This type of fatigue can be eliminated by a nutritious meal and pep talk in the locker room during the sports interval. There are many instances when athletes enter the locker room feeling tired and defeated, and then a good snack followed by their coach's motivational speech drastically uplifts their performance.

3. Psychological fatigue:

Psychological, emotional, and social factors from an athlete's competition, team, school, work, finances, family, and friends can all add up very fast, leaving the athlete mentally drained and desperate.

This can manifest as a loss in self-confidence or self-esteem or change in attitude or behavior.

Psychological fatigue need not present with muscle fatigue; instead it may present as a reduced attention span and wakefulness (i.e., somnolence and loss of drive).

In psychology this decreased attention span is termed *ego depletion*, because the capacity to self-regulate activities is depleted.

In some cases the athlete may be absentminded (due to reduced awareness) and lose focus during tasks that require constant concentration. In such cases where psychological fatigue is suspected, a psychological objective cognitive test should reveal any associated neuro-cognitive deficits.

Assessment of psychological fatigue:

Many methods of assessment have been developed to scale the degrees of mental fatigue. Hacker and Richter (1994) have accomplished most of the significant work in this field. The scaling for mental/psychological fatigue has been developed based on the individual's capacity to cope with behavioral decrements:

Level 1: *Optimal and efficient performance*: no symptoms of decrement in performance, mood, and activation level.

Level 2: *Complete compensation characterized by increased peripheral psycho-physiological activation* (e.g., measurement shown by electromyogram for finger muscles), perception of increased mental effort required to complete tasks, increased variability in performance criteria.

Level 3: *Labile compensation additional to that described in level 2*: a feeling of fatigue, and action slips, increasing (compensatory) psycho-physiological activity in central indicators, heart rate, and blood pressure.

Level 4: *Reduced efficiency additional to that described in level 3*: decrease in performance criteria.

Level 5: *Yet further functional disturbances*: instances of conflicts in social relationships and at workplace; symptoms of clinical fatigue such as feelings of exhaustion and decreased quality of sleep.

4. Environmental/ travel fatigue:

The following factors can add up quickly and lead to fatigue:

Extended travel periods. Extended periods of travel require the athlete to be seated in a stationary position; this reduces blood flow and lymphatic circulation to various parts of the body and leaves the athlete feeling dull.

Poor exposure to natural light. During periods of travel or training, the athlete may stay indoors for extended periods of time. Lack of exposure to natural sunlight can reduce the production of melatonin, thereby producing a low mood and lethargy. Dim lighting is also known to produce fatigue.

Environmental pollution. This can include sound and air pollution; it may be connected with extended periods of travel in traffic or training in a noisy environment. These noises put the person in a fight-or-flight mode, causing them to function in a state of high alertness, as if the body was facing an imminent threat from the environment.

The body reacts to this situation by producing tiny amounts of cortisol and adrenaline; over the long term, this phenomenon can weaken athletes' immune systems and ultimately leave them exhausted by the end of the season.

Tips to counter sound pollution: using earplugs or playing soft background music can prove to be beneficial in such circumstances.

Tips to counter air pollution: use carbon-based face masks for bicycle commuting in pollen-infected areas and for cutting down the pollutants sucked into the lungs in heavy traffic regions. These masks can also be used to filter out large amounts of particulate matter from the air during long-distance runs.

Ergonomics of travel. Depending on the nature of travel, the seating and stay arrangements encountered during travel may not be ergonomic or conducive for optimal recovery. Ergonomic seating prevents slumped posture and bad breathing, which can lead to fatigue.

An ideal ergonomic position would be one that provides adequate support to the lumbar region and allows adjustable seats, so that the feet can be rested flat on the floor with the thighs parallel to the ground. This allows the athlete to breathe comfortably. A frequent change in posture along with regular standing, walking, and stretching will help provide better body circulation and prevent cramps during travel.

Temperature. A training room that is too warm can quickly raise the core temperature of athletes' bodies and cause them to feel tired very quickly. Other factors such as humidity can also affect athletes' perspiration rates and cause them to lose body fluids very quickly.

Jet lag. Jet lag can be a major factor that can easily cause fatigue; since the athletes sleep and wake times are impacted significantly, it's important to note that even a two-hour delay in sleep due to jet lag can impact athletes' recovery after heavy training.

This factor should be considered before an athlete embarks upon international competitions; a good strategy would be to arrive a few days early at the international training venue, so the athlete's body gets enough time to adjust to the change in circadian rhythm.

Other environmental and travel factors that can impact the fatigue and recovery patterns of athletes include changes in elevation, climate changes (changes in air pressure), inconsistent wake-up times, changing meal times, and dehydration.

Stress:

What is stress?

According to the biopsychological stress model by Janke and Wolffgramm (1995), stress is an unspecific reaction-oriented syndrome that is characterized by a deviation from the biological homeostatic state. Any deviation from the normal balance in life can be considered as stress.

There are two main types of stress: eustress and distress.

- Eustress is a term coined by endocrinologist Hans Selye. Eustress is defined in the model of Richard Lazarus (1974) as stress that is healthy, or gives one a feeling of fulfillment or other positive feelings. Eustress is a process of exploring potential gains. It is defined as a good type of stress that stems from the challenge of a pleasant activity.

- This type of stress is experienced by all athletes; it helps the athlete get motivated and pumped up before a performance.

- Eustress can be experienced whenever we push our limits and strive to achieve greater heights. This type of stress allows us to grow and push beyond our usual limitations.

- Distress is defined as the bad type of stress that arises when you must adapt to negative demands. Distress is an unexpected and unwelcome type of stress. In this situation athletes may be unable to adapt completely to the stressors and their resulting stress and may display maladaptive behaviors such as inappropriate modes of social interaction (e.g., aggression, passivity, or withdrawal).

Athletes need to be able to differentiate between the two types of stress and become self-aware. In the upcoming section, we will look at the situations and triggers that can lead to distress.

What are the potential stressors in an athlete's life?

Any event or situation the individual perceives as a threat or challenge can be considered a stressor. The stressor may be physical or psychological; how well the athlete copes with and reacts to the stressor determines the athlete's overall state of mind and well-being.

If athletes have poor coping mechanisms or react poorly to sudden critical situations, then their bodies are likely to produce cortisol and adrenaline, which can upset their metabolism and make them prone to psychological and physical problems.

Stressors can be classified into three main categories:

1. Crises/catastrophes

2. Major life events

3. Daily hassles/ microstressors

Crises/catastrophes:

This is a situation where the athlete's life has been impacted by an unpredictable or unforeseen event. Examples of such stressors include natural disasters, earthquakes, hurricanes, major floods, and wars.

Studies conducted at the University of Stanford have revealed that natural catastrophes cause a significant increase in stress levels experienced by the affected.

Going through such catastrophes can cause athletes to feel immense pressure; their career takes a side seat, and they watch as helpless spectators.

Major life events:

Major life events cause a significant change in lifestyle or relationships. Examples of such major life events can include

- Divorce,

- Change in sporting environment/team,

- Breakup,

- Marriage,

- New college,

- New part-time job,

- Major financial loss,

- Birth of a child, or

- Loss of a loved one.

Research has shown that major life events can have a great impact on life, especially when they are negative. The impact of negative major life events is felt only over the long term, and the short-term effects are usually negligible. Chronic events that have created stress in the past can manifest as illnesses later on in life.

Free radicals create oxidative stress. Each cell in our bodies is sur-rounded by a membrane made up of high-molecular-weight unsaturated fatty-acid molecules called phospholipids. When the body does not have enough natural antioxidants to protect it from the reactive, oxygen-based free radicals that we produce as a by-product of breathing (collectively known as reactive oxygen species, or ROS), these phospholipids (as well as proteins and DNA) can be attacked by the excess free radicals, resulting in a condition we call oxidative stress.

Many diseases, as well as exposures to toxins, are known to cause oxidative stress; these can include heart disease, cancer, and autoimmune and neurodegenerative diseases (M. Trevisan, *American Journal of Epidemiology* 2001).

Daily hassles/microstressors:

Microstressors are events that create stress in everyday life. These can include minor conflicts and disturbances. Examples of such situations include

- Traffic jams,

- Workplace conflicts,

- Daily annoyances,

- Unexpected cancellations/ delays, and

- Making decisions.

Why is it important to handle stress?

In *Stress and Performance in Sport*, author Graham Jones writes, "Sports performance is not simply a product of physiological (for example stress and fitness) and biomechanical (for example technique factors) but psychological factors also play a crucial role in determining performance" (New York: John Wiley and Sons, 1990).

We are all aware of the fact that stress can decrease an athlete's performance; let's have a quick look at how stress can impact the athlete physically and why it is important to eliminate stress in its early stages.

It's vital to understand that pre-game jitters or nervousness on the morning of the big game is very normal in a competitive situation; the athlete's preparation is about to be put to the test, and this can create feelings of fight or flight; the athlete may experience loss of appetite or loss of sleep prior to the night of the big competition. This is seen especially in situations where the athlete has a lot on the line and needs to give a big performance.

However, the presence of chronic stress can have a significant impact on performance.

During periods of stress, our body produces two harmful chemicals: cortisol and adrenaline. These chemicals can affect all the body's systems and cause symptoms of wear and tear in otherwise fit athletes.

Cortisol is produced by the adrenal glands, located on top of the kidneys; this hormone has a powerful effect on the body. The major role of cortisol is to mobilize your body and generate quick fuel during stressful situations. Cortisol increases blood sugar levels over the short term and helps the athlete become more alert and energetic. However, if the secretion of cortisol is prolonged, it can affect mental function and alertness (Taverniers 2010).

Cortisol also produces a strong immunosuppressive effect on the body; this delays healing and recovery after an athletic performance. The levels of adrenaline also increase in conjunction with cortisol; this further provokes the fight-or-flight response and upsets the psychology of the athlete.

Studies conducted by Nippert et al. in 2008 clearly demonstrate that psychosocial stressors such as personality, history of stressors, and life-event stress can influence injury occurrence. After injury, those same factors plus athletic identity, self-esteem, and significant others—such as parents, coaches, and teammates—can affect injury response, recovery, and subsequent sport performance. [13]

Top ten harmful syndromes created by stress:

1) Loss of athletic body shape

Increased levels of cortisol can produce a catabolic state in athletes; during this catabolic state, the athlete loses lean muscle mass and starts storing fat. These effects start kicking into full force when the athlete does not consume adequate calories. If there are periods without caloric consumption when the athlete has a high demand for them, the body will then go into a catabolic state.

Cortisol is also known to promote central obesity; that is, it causes fat to accumulate in the central part of the body. This can be very detrimental to the athlete's performance, because loss of lean muscle and accumulation of fat in the central region reduces the athlete's performance.

2) Stress harms the immune system

Our body has a natural, inbuilt capacity to produce T cells and fight off any infectious agents. However, whenever a person experiences stress, the associated increase in cortisol levels blocks off the multiplication of cells and thereby reduces the body's ability to defend itself against infectious agents such as bacteria and viruses.

This makes the athlete more prone to fatigue, infections, and lethargy.

Stress is also known to produce a decrease in levels of testosterone, estrogen, and progesterone. Such decreased levels of testosterone can further impact the recovery rate in males, and decreased levels of estrogen and progesterone slows down recovery in females.

3) Stress can destabilize blood pressure by making the blood vessels more sensitive to adrenaline and by blocking potassium from escaping the blood vessels.

Whenever athletes prepare for a performance, their bodies produce adrenaline; blood vessels that are more sensitive to adrenaline can create sudden fluctuations of blood pressure (BP) in the athlete.

Chronically high blood pressure is especially damaging to our blood vessels, wearing and tearing them down quicker than usual. Due to the intense pressure, the otherwise smooth linings in the interior of our blood vessels suffer microscopic tears and become rough and uneven.

The tiny depressions on the inside of our vessels trigger the body's inflammatory response, which attempts to repair the tears. A flurry of pro-inflammatory cells and hormones, together with other fatty nutrients such as cholesterol, begin to flood the injury sites.

4) Stress can lower the athlete's intelligence. Studies have revealed that chronic exposure to cortisol can cause damage and death of cells in the hippocampus. Unfortunately this is the part of the brain that is responsible for storing memory and learned behavior. Chronic stress can impair the athlete's ability to learn and memorize critical bits of information and make judgments.

5) Stress has been directly linked to low mood. Cortisol is directly related to an increased incidence of anxiety and depression.

6) Stress leads to many metabolic disorders: cortisol is the prime culprit behind development of several metabolic disorders, which include digestive disorders, acidity in the stomach, and diabetes mellitus type II. Cortisol blocks the function of insulin in the body; this leads to an increased level of blood sugar and predisposes to diabetes.

Increased levels of acidity in the stomach can lead to stomach ulcers and digestive disorders in the gut.

7) Cortisol can weaken the reproductive system and lead to loss of libido and impotency. This can create trouble in relationships.

8) Stress directly affects appetite control and satiety: many research studies have revealed that stress can cause increased food cravings and cause the athlete to drink and eat more than usual.

9) Cortisol can predispose to easy fractures: it's known to be an osteolytic agent, reducing the rate of bone regeneration and bone formation. This causes loss of calcium from the bones and predisposes to easy fractures.

As stress continues to persist, the athlete may become prone to experiencing stress fractures.

10) Relationship between stress and cancer: a direct relationship between psychological stress and the development of cancer has not been scientifically proven; however, research scientists from the National Cancer Institute have suggested that psychological factors may affect cancer progression (increase in tumor size or spread of cancer in the body) in patients who have the disease.

Other effects of stress: some athletes may experience reduced exercise capacity and feel breathy very early during the training session. Some women may complain of amenorrhea.

The effects described above are related mostly to cortisol. The other major hormone produced during stress is adrenaline. Increased levels of adrenaline are directly related to palpitations in the chest, sensations of panic, uneasiness, anxiety, increased heart rate, restlessness, tremors in the limbs, increased blood pressure, difficulty in breathing, and heart arrhythmia and damage.

Studies by Ronsen et al. (2002) have shown that introducing recovery time between training sessions can significantly reduce cortisol levels and promote recovery. Further use of adaptogens and rhodiola may help in reducing cortisol levels and improve the body's response to stress. [14]

However, just managing levels of cortisol will not solve the problem. The approach needs to be multifaceted; it needs to start with a complete psychological evaluation of stressors and analysis of the nutrition, training, and recovery schedules of the athlete.

How can we evaluate levels of stress in an athlete?

Stress may manifest with emotional, physical, cognitive, or behavioral signs and symptoms.

Whenever athletes suffers from stress, they may exhibit poor judgment, complain about lack of confidence, appear to be worrying excessively, show signs of irritability and agitation, find it difficult to relax, and complain of loneliness or depression.

Stress may manifest with physical symptoms such as aches and pains in the muscles, acne, chest pain, dizziness, diarrhea or constipation, nausea, changes in appetite, and sleep disturbance.

Behaviorally the athlete may procrastinate before training, neglect responsibilities, and increase consumption of alcohol, nicotine, or other drugs.

Since all the symptoms cannot be quantified subjectively, we need to rely on a more concrete scale to measure stress levels in athletes.

The most commonly used scale to measure stress was developed by psychiatrists Thomas Holmes and Richard Rahe. This is known as the Social Readjustment Rating Scale, or SRRS, or Holmes and Rahe Stress Scale; it contains a comprehensive list of forty-three events that can cause stress.

Each stressful event is given a stress score (known as life-change units) in the Richard Rahe scale; to estimate the amount of stress an athlete faces in a lifetime, the athlete needs to take the test and tick the situations they currently face.

A score of more than 300 means implies that the individual faces a high risk for illness, a score between 150 and 299 means risk of illness is moderate, and a score under 150 means that individual has only a slight risk of illness.

This test helps in deciding the type of intervention required for the player. For example, an athlete with a very high stress score may need a psychologist's help. The test is a useful tool to estimate the well-being of an athlete at any given point and plan appropriate management. If left unattended, stress can be expressed as anxiety, anger, and changes in immune function.

The Richard Rahe scale:

Life event	Life change units
Death of a spouse	100
Divorce	73
Marital separation	65
Imprisonment	63
Death of a close family member	63
Personal injury or illness	53
Marriage	50
Dismissal from work	47
Marital reconciliation	45
Retirement	45
Change in health of family member	44
Pregnancy	40
Sexual difficulties	39
Gain a new family member	39
Business readjustment	39
Change in financial state	38
Death of a close friend	37
Change to different line of work	36
Change in frequency of arguments	35
Major mortgage	32
Foreclosure of mortgage or loan	30
Change in responsibilities at work	29
Child leaving home	29
Trouble with in-laws	29
Outstanding personal achievement	28
Spouse starts or stops work	26
Begin or end school	26

Life event	Life change units
Change in living conditions	25
Revision of personal habits	24
Trouble with boss	23
Change in working hours or conditions	20
Change in residence	20
Change in schools	20
Change in recreation	19
Change in church activities	19
Change in social activities	18
Minor mortgage or loan	17
Change in sleeping habits	16
Change in number of family reunions	15
Change in eating habits	14
Vacation	13
Minor violation of law	10

Total score = _____

Date: _____

Remarks: _____

_____

_____

_____

_____

Illness:

The typical forms of illness that athletes experience are usually viral infections related to the upper respiratory tract. Among these infections, the common cold the most frequent form of viral illness. Illness due to influenza virus may also be seen in athletes, although it is less common.

Epstein-Barr virus causes glandular fever or infectious mononucleosis in young athletes and teenage competitors; it's estimated that nearly 70 to 90 percent of athletes come in contact with Epstein-Barr virus at some point during their training and competition. [15]

Since the immune system of most young athletes is very strong, they are able to fight off the infection; however, a small number of athletes may exhibit signs of glandular fever, which includes fatigue, generalized weakness, and swollen glands. In case of viral illness, the general signs include

- Sore throat,

- Headache,

- Nausea,

- Diarrhea,

- Sneezing,

- Spike in fatigue, and

- Increase in morning heart rate.

After an Epstein-Barr virus infection, the athlete may need several weeks or even months for complete recovery.

Other forms of illness seen in athletes include the following:

- *Fungal infections*—tinea versicolor infection: This is a fungal infection that appears as small, itchy flat spots on the skin. In some cases the spots may blend into a big patchy area. The spots are usually flaky. This infection is seen during the summer season, especially when the climate is hot and humid. It is usually seen in the upper chest, back, or upper arms, and is more likely to be seen in individuals with oily skin. A tinea versicolor infection is not contagious. A diagnosis of this infection is made by studying the skin-scrape sample with a KOH test. Treatment is via a topical antifungal shampoo or solution.

- *Intertrigo*—yeast infection in skin folds: a reddish brown rash seen between the skin folds. It may be seen in the armpits or in skin folds in the genital region.

- *Ringworm*, also known as tinea corporis, causes a fungal infection that lives and multiplies on the top layer of the skin and hair. Ringworm infection typically presents as a very itchy rash. It commonly appears in a pattern similar to a ring, but not always. In a few cases, it may just present as a red, itchy rash.

- It's important to note that the ringworm infection is highly contagious. It spreads via skin contact and can be contracted from another person or an animal. This organism is usually found in warm and moist areas, such as swimming pools, locker rooms, and moist skin folds. It may also spread through shared items in the locker room such as towels, sports equipment, and clothing items.

- *Athlete's foot* (fungal infection with tinea pedis) is a commonly seen fungal infection, and it can be prevented by washing the feet regularly and taking measures to dry the feet properly (especially between the toes), wearing sandals in warm weather, and using bathing slippers in public bathrooms.

- *Jock itch* (fungal infection with tinea cruris): This infection appears as a red and itchy rash in the groin region. The best way to prevent this rash from appearing is by showering immediately after a sports activity and using dry cotton briefs after the shower.

- *Parasites*: Encountered especially during travel.

- *Allergies or asthma* induced by exercise may be seen increasingly during the spring season, when the pollen count in the atmosphere is very high.

Whenever an athlete presents with signs of illness, it's a good strategy to be safe rather than sorry; the best policy would be to refer the athlete to a physician for a proper examination and blood tests if necessary; this will help the athlete understand the symptoms of illness at a very early stage and help him or her take extra precautions to avoid illness during the next few training sessions; such enhanced precautionary measures help keep athletes focused on their recovery process and keeps everybody on the same page.

Important factors to consider:

An athlete who is recovering from an illness may be a silent carrier of the disease; depending on the nature of the illness, it may spread from athlete to athlete.

The common modes of disease transmission include the following:

Athlete to athlete. Chances of infection via contact sport are very high for professionals training in sports such as martial arts, football, wrestling, professional fighting, boxing, rugby, basketball, field hockey, and volleyball, due to direct skin-to-skin contact.

- Hand-shaking: direct transmission of communicable diseases.

- Closed environment: transmission of airborne and respiratory-tract infections.

Transmission via air. Coughing or sneezing releases droplets of mucus secretions into the air; these droplets have the potential to spread the infection quickly. If the co-athlete is within three feet of the infected person, there's a very high chance of transmission of infection. Droplets usually contain highly contagious germs and have more potential to cause infection than direct contact.

Almost all respiratory infections are spread via droplet transmission: some of the common diseases spread this way are pneumonia, streptococcus throat infection, meningeal (brain) infections, upper-respiratory-tract infections, and ear infections.

Fungi and parasites cannot be transmitted via droplet infection.

Spread of infection in the training area. *Esherichia coli* bacteria commonly spread via hand contact; this commonly happens whenever athletes are infected and do not wash their hands after using the bathroom. Organisms that cause gastroenteritis also spread when an athlete consumes food or snacks without hand-washing. The most common organism that causes food poisoning and gut infections is salmonella; this infection can spread rapidly to other individuals.

Transmission through indirect contact. This occurs mostly through an intermediate object such as a door knob or training equipment. The germs spread over the intermediate object whenever the athlete uses the object. Some forms of bacteria and fungi are cosmopolitan and survive in almost any environment, including inanimate objects. Viruses can also survive on inanimate objects but only for a short term. If healthy individuals touch these objects, they run the risk of catching the illness. The most common illnesses spread through indirect contact are the common cold (rhinovirus) and stomach flu.

Transmission through water. Disease is very often caused by contaminated drinking water and uncooked foods. *E. coli* is one of the most common organisms present in uncooked foods, and it is responsible for food poisoning. Municipal water provided by government agencies goes through a thorough purification process before it reaches the consumer; however, water sourced from private wells and private agencies may be contaminated due to their storage systems; this water carries a great potential for causing illness. Special attention should be paid to water during travel and cross-country competitions. Athletes should be warned not to consume any water handed by spectators or strangers.

Transmission via recreational swimming pools. During cross-country competitions the athletes may come across many opportunities to take part in water sports and water-based recreational activities that can take place in spas, pools, lakes, rivers, and so on; natural water resources often carry the risk of being contaminated by animal waste, fungus, chemicals, or sewage. Human or animal contamination can pollute the water with germs such as *E. coli* and *Giardia*. The Centers for Disease Control has reported many outbreaks of diarrhea, respiratory infections, gastrointestinal infections, skin diseases, and eye, ear, and wound infections originating from these water resources.

While using disinfectants such as chlorine and other special disinfectants may kill germs, certain parasites such as *Cryptosporidium* are resistant to disinfectants. *Cryptosporidium* is currently the leading cause for recreational water illness (RWI). Since natural water resources such as lakes and streams cannot be chlorinated, they carry a higher chance of infection when compared to indoor water recreation available at spas and resorts.

Cross-infection within the patient:

- Rubbing eyes: transmission of bacterial and fungal infections to the eyes.

- Picking nose: transmission of bacterial and fungal infections to the nose.

- Biting nails: transmission of fungal infections to the tongue (The infectious agent is lodged within the fingernail after scratching.)

Recovery regimen and training schedule:

The most important factor for athletes and trainers is the time lost due to illness and the confusion regarding when the athlete should return to training and at what intensity the athlete should be training.

The time allotted for recovery will primarily depend on the severity of illness, the cause of illness, and the rate of recovery exhibited by the athlete.

The Australian Institute of Sport (Pyne et al. 1995; Young 1999) developed a simple, three-step approach to help athletes, trainers, and physicians make a decision regarding the time allotted for recovery.

The three most important elements to be considered before an athlete returns to training are

1) Frequency of training sessions,

2) Duration of training, and

3) Intensity of training expected from the athlete.

The primary objective of the athlete in resuming training after the break is to start slowly and then gradually increase the frequency (number) of training sessions.

Once the athlete adapts to the frequency of training, the next step would be to methodically increase the duration of each training session.

After the second step has been achieved—that is, after the athlete has started training at the optimal frequency and is able to maintain stamina for the optimal length of time—the next step would be to increase the intensity of training.

This three-step process helps the athlete to return to an optimal level of training after a period of illness.

The duration of this process may vary from a few days (in case of mild illness) to a few weeks (in case of moderate illness) or a few months (severe illness.)

The recommended length and intensity of training during the initial stages of training is around twenty to thirty minutes of low-intensity aerobic exercise.

This may be carried out as a separate (individual) training session away from the normal training group. It is ideal to maintain a light to moderate intensity of exercise during these sessions; the heart rate should be approximately 60 to 70 percent of the athlete's maximum heart rate.

For example, the target heart rate would be in the range of 120–140 bpm for an athlete whose maximum heart rate is 200 bpm.

If the athlete is able to endure the training sessions and recover well after the training session, then she or he may carry out a similar session the following day. When the athlete has achieved enough fitness to train and recover completely over many consecutive days, the coach may increase the training frequency to two times per day and sustain that frequency of training for the next few days.

Variations of training cycles:

If the nature of illness is not very severe, the trainer may choose to start with a single session of training on the first and second day, then move up to two sessions on the third day, and finally come down to a single session on day four.

The cycle can be repeated over the next few days.

If the nature of illness is moderate or severe, than the trainer may choose to start with a single session of training on the first day, then follow it up with one day of rest.

The cycle can be repeated over the next few days.

The duration of training sessions mostly depends on the previous training history and fitness of the athlete.

An athlete who had a very high level of fitness prior to the illness and missed training sessions only for one or two days due to mild illness can increase the volume (duration) of exercise considerably fast;

however, if an athlete has missed many days of practice due to illness or has been away from training for many months due to severe illness, that athlete will need a few weeks to resume his or her full volume of practice.

The duration of rehabilitation should be similar to the amount of time lost due to illness. For instance, a one-week rehabilitation plan may be adequate for an athlete who has missed training for one week due to illness.

Intensity of practice and training needs to be increased as a last step of rehabilitation. It is not advisable to increase the intensity of exercise first; this is a typical mistake among trainers. Sudden increments of training and high-intensity workouts can weaken the immune system and make the athlete prone to reinfection.

Tiny, 5–10 percent increments in intensity of training always facilitate health recovery.

Alternating periods of low- and high-intensity exercise with adequate time for recovery helps the athlete recover faster and train at optimal levels. It's also beneficial to allow more recovery time during high-intensity training sessions.

For example, if an athlete takes a thirty-second break between circuit training sessions, then that athlete may be allowed to take a sixty- to ninety-second break between circuit training sessions during the rehabilitation.

The athlete needs to be educated about the importance of maintaining awareness during recovery and must be trained to observe the signs of illness and recovery.

A training diary is a very helpful tool in monitoring the health and wellness of a recovering athlete. The most important details that need to be noted during periods of recovery are as follows:

1) Levels of performance reached during training—check if the athlete is able to reach and maintain performance at previous levels (prior to illness).

2) Feelings of tiredness or weakness.

3) Symptoms such as heavy-headedness, flulike symptoms, pains and aches, or fever.

4) Heart-rate monitoring: before, during, and after exercise compared with heart rates prior to illness.

5) Changes in body weight and body fat percentage.

6) Recovery time after a training session.

7) Training hangover and improper recovery the next day after a training session.

8) Irritability—feeling low or anxious over the last few days.

9) Apprehension, self-doubt, and feelings of guilt.

It is ideal for the athlete and coach to be monitoring this diary on a frequent basis during the period of rehabilitation. This will ease a lot of pressure and stress for both the athlete and the trainer.

During the recovery period, the coach and the athlete may observe some signs of relapse; this is part of a normal rehabilitation process. If the coach feels that the symptoms continue to persist or recur frequently despite reduced levels of training, then it would be beneficial to get a checkup and treatment at a doctor's clinic.

It's also important to note that eating habits and hydration can play a major role in the recovery process; therefore, it is important to consume a diet that strengthens the immunity and facilitates recovery.

Precautions to prevent illness:

In order to prevent transmission of a disease agent during training sessions, the following precautions must be taken.

Athletes should be educated about the infective potential of body substances such as blood, secretions (except sweat), body fluids, wounds, and mucous membranes and how these substances can act as potential vehicles for transmission of infectious agents.

The following standard precautions must be taken to prevent cross-infection among athletes:

1) The coach or trainer needs to always wear gloves before touching open skin, body secretions, or mucous membranes of athletes.

2) Soap and hot water should be used to wash hands thoroughly after contact with the above-mentioned body substances (even if gloves have been used).

3) All the training surfaces that can act as indirect sources of transmission must be cleaned with diluted bleach (preferably a 10-percent solution); this helps in cleaning out all the infectious organisms, including MRSA.

4) Disinfect and cover all wounds before the athlete enters the field of play.

In case of the skin injury or abrasion on the playing ground, it is advisable to remove the athlete from the field of play and provide medical attention, so that the injured area is clean and sealed with bandages; this prevents player infection and the leakage of body fluids on the field.

Equipment disinfection:

For efficient prevention of disease transmission, the training and sports equipment must be cleaned and sterilized whenever possible.

As discussed earlier, training equipment can serve as a source of indirect transmission. In many cases research conducted on training facilities has revealed presence of methicillin-resistant *Staphylococcus aureus* (MRSA—a dangerous, drug-resistant bacteria) and pseudomonas on taping gel and whirlpool facilities. These organisms have been linked to many infectious outbreaks at training centers.

Complete guidelines for regular disinfection and hygienic maintenance of saunas, ice machines, whirlpools, and swimming pools can be obtained from the Occupational Safety and Health Administration (OSHA), USA.

According to disinfection guidelines, a diluted 10-percent bleach solution (nine parts water to one part bleach) is effective in disinfecting training equipment and floors.

Educating the athlete: Prevention of cross-infection within the athlete:

The athlete must be advised to keep fingernails short.

The athlete needs to be educated about hygiene.

The athlete needs to be educated about the modes of disease transmission.

Encourage athletes to maintain their own sets of clothes: advise them to keep a pack of an extra set of clean clothes, towels, flip-flops (to wear in the bathroom), and toiletries. A hygiene checklist must always include the maintenance of a personal set of gym clothes and accessories and frequent use of laundry service.

Athletes must be taught the proper technique for hand hygiene:

Proper hand-washing is highly effective in reducing illnesses and transmission of microbes. The protocol recommended by the Mayo Clinic and the Association for Professionals in Infection Control and Epidemiology is as follows:

1) Turn on running water, and wet your hands thoroughly (including your palms up to the wrists).

2) Use the liquid-soap dispenser and squeeze a generous amount of liquid soap into your hands.

3) Work up a good lather by vigorously rubbing your hands together for about fifteen seconds.

4) Make sure the lather reaches all parts of your hands, which include your palms, spaces between the fingers, back of your hands, your fingernail crevices, and your wrists.

5) Rinse your hands under the water, and make sure all the areas of your hands are cleaned thoroughly.

6) Dry your hands using an air blower/dryer or paper dryer.

7) The faucet of the tap and the doorknob of the bathroom can act as indirect carriers of infections; hence it would be safe to use a paper tissue to turn off the faucet of the tap and open the doorknob. It is also important to use a paper towel to turn on/off taps, open doors, and flush toilets when using a public restroom.

8) If the hand-washing facilities are not ideal for proper hand-washing, then the athlete may choose to use an alcohol-based hand sanitizer. The process of hand cleaning is similar to that of a regular hand wash: athletes are advised to squeeze a generous amount of hand sanitizer into their hands and ensure that all surfaces of the hands are thoroughly covered, including the back of the hands and the wrist. The cleaning process must be thorough and should take up to thirty seconds.

9) Frequent hand-washing with sanitizer must be encouraged in all athletes.

10) Chlorhexidine soap is known to be useful for reducing transmission of MRSA infections. (MRSA stands for methicillin-resistant *Staphylococcus aureus*; it is a *Staphylococcus* bacteria that spreads by touching among athletes who share items such as towels and razors. The infection may manifest with chest pain, respiratory infections, or allergic symptoms; the infection is resistant to first-line antibiotics such as methicillin and requires stronger and expensive antibiotics, and therefore it is known as methicillin-resistant Staphylococcus aureus, or MRSA.)

Formula for simple disinfectant to clean the gym and workout area: to 1 gallon of clean water in a bucket, mix 1/4 cup of household bleach; this solution can be used for disinfection and wiping gym surfaces.

*It's important to note that disinfectants can irritate the lungs, skin, and eyes.

General instructions to avoid disease transmission via contact sport:

- Try to avoid contact with other athlete's wounds, blood, sweat, or bandages.

- Ask the other athlete to clean up any body secretions and cover wounds cleanly before engaging in contact sport.

- Ensure all cuts and scrapes are cleanly covered with a bandage until the healing process is complete.

- Make sure protocols are in place to wipe and clean gym equipment before and after use.

- Place stickers in the training rooms to discourage sharing of any clothes, training items, or towels.

- It's a good habit to shower immediately after exercise whenever possible; if immediate showering is not an option, then you may consider cleaning all body sweat thoroughly with a towel and changing into a clean set of clothes.

- The workout gear must be placed in a separate plastic bag and handed over for immediate wash.

- Ensure that all the workout clothes are washed and dried after each workout.

Transmission control during sport:

Use a fist bump instead of a handshake: a handshake is generally used among friends and athletes as a form of greeting or as a gesture of a job well done.

The handshake may serve as a vehicle to transfer of germs, viruses, bacteria, and other microbes.

Since it's almost impossible to estimate what the other person has touched prior to the handshake, bumping a closed fist with another athlete offers a good alternative to a vigorous handshake; this can serve as an easy way to prevent the spread of infection.

Cough into an elbow instead of hands: it is estimated that a single sneeze produces nearly forty thousand droplets of moisture and many millions of germs; the average speed of a forceful sneeze is between 80 mph and 100 mph, and it can propel the germ particles up to a distance of thirty-two feet.

Another deadly pandemic that can be transported via a sneeze is the H5N1 infection; when a person acquires this infection over an already existing influenza infection, it can prove to be deadly.

The typical advice of covering the nose and mouth during a sneeze can actually facilitate the spread of disease, because viruses can be readily transferred via touch.

The use of regular-sized tissues to cover the nose and mouth area during sneezing may not be effective, since it allows air leakage. Only men's-size tissues have been found to be effective to adequately absorb the germ particles in a sneeze.

Coughing and sneezing into the crook of the elbow has been found to be effective in minimizing the spread of germs. Hence athletes must be advised to cough or sneeze into their elbow crooks.

Health protection during travel:

Extensive country-specific health information and travel recommendations can be obtained from the official CDC website.

It provides information for travelers about the specific diseases pertaining to each region; the database covers more than one hundred travel-related diseases and lists country-specific information, vaccines, and travel tips.

For country-specific information, go to http://wwwnc.cdc.gov/travel/destinations/list.htm.

For disease-specific information, go to http://wwwnc.cdc.gov/travel/page/diseases.htm.

It is also important for the athlete to actively report all the details of travel to the doctor, because the doctor may not be actively looking for uncommon infections (e.g., protozoan infection) and may miss out on making an accurate diagnosis.

References:

(1)   Allen and Westerblad 2001.

(2)   Lorist et al. 2002.

(3)   Davis et al. 2003.

(4)   Edgley and Winter 2004.

(5)   Kallenberget al. 2007.

(6)   St. Clair Gibson et al. 2003.

(7)   Bigland-Ritchie and Woods.1984; Søgaard et al. 2006.

(8)   Vøllestad, N. K. *J Neurosci Methods*. 1997. 74(2):219–27.

(9)   Hicks, Kent-Braun, and Ditor 2001.

(10) Hicks, Kent-Braun, and Ditor 2001.

(11) Roger et al. *J Physiol* 586.1 (2008) pp. 11–23.

(12) Fitts 1994.

(13) *Phys Med RehabilClin N Am.* 2008.19(2):399–418, x. doi: 10.1016/j.pmr.2007.12.003.

(14) Olsson 2009, Parnossian 2009, Zhang 2009.

(15) Pyne, D. B., Gray, A. B., and McDonald, W. A. 1995. "Exercise, training, and immunity." In *Textbook of Science and Medicine in Sport.* J. Bloomfield, P. Fricker, and K. Fitch (eds.) Melbourne: Blackwell Science, pp. 602–15. http://www.ausport.gov.au/sportscoachmag/program_management2/how_to_manage_the_return_to_training_after_illness

The Second Pillar of Recovery

Rest

The Second Pillar of Recovery: Rest

REST IS MANDATORY FOR A HEALTHY LIFESTYLE; IT refreshes the body and mind, rejuvenates mood, and enhances learning and memory. Lack of rest can worsen the immune system and stress levels and ultimately lead to poor mood and poor performance.

Let's look at the top seven reasons to get enough rest:

1) *Immunity:* It's been found that sleep deprivation inhibits the activity of body's killer T cells. The cells help fight off infection; however, in the absence of proper sleep, they are unable to function at their optimum levels. Good sleep also helps fight cancer-inducing agents.

2) *Better circulation:* Improper sleep has been linked to increased levels of stress hormones, blood pressure, and irregular heartbeat. Getting enough rest and sleep helps support cardiovascular health.

3) *Mental health:* Poor rest has been associated with increased levels of cortisol and adrenaline, which in turn can lead to anger, frustration, poor focus, and bad moods.

4) *Alertness:* It's been shown that people who do not get adequate sleep and rest have poor response times and are prone to make errors in judgment and strategy.

5) *Procrastination:* Sleep debt has been associated with a greater tendency to feel sleepy and have high levels of procrastination and low motivation. This causes the athlete to avoid training routines and protocols.

6) *Learning and memory:* People who are sleep-deprived are unable to learn new information and store it in their long-term memory (poor memory consolidation). Studies have revealed that learning and memory improve after adequate rest.

7) *Metabolism and fitness:* Sleep affects the way our body metabolizes stored carbohydrates. When the athlete does not get adequate rest or sleep, the body perceives a threat and starts storing fat for long-term use.

Research studies on sleep:

Studies carried out by Eve Van Cauter, PhD, from the University of Chicago Medical School have revealed the links between sleep, cortisol, and glucose metabolism.

The effects of three different durations of sleep were tested in men aged eighteen to twenty-seven. The men were allowed to sleep eight hours per night for the first three nights, four hours per night for the next six nights, and twelve hours per night for the last seven nights.

Tests revealed that the glucose was metabolized least efficiently and cortisol levels were at their highest during periods of sleep deprivation (four hours of sleep per night).

Other studies revealed that just one week of sleep restriction in young, healthy males caused significant disturbances in glucose metabolism, decreased glycogen synthesis, decreased activity of growth hormone, and disturbance of other body functions.

The young men also reported decreased aerobic endurance and higher ratings of perceived exertion.

Optimal levels of sleep recommended for athletes:

The amount of rest required by athletes varies according to their levels of activity and physical demands; the need for sleep and rest varies during resting periods (long training breaks) and periods of intensive exercise.

Amount of sleep required during resting periods (long training breaks):

Excess sleep (more than eight hours) is not necessarily a good thing.

According Dr. Daniel Kripke (Scripps Clinic Sleep Center, La Jolla, California), who studied the sleep habits of more than one million people in the US, people who sleep between 6.5 hrs. and 7.5 hrs. enjoy the best health. People who sleep less than 6.5 hrs. or more than 8 hrs. have higher rates of sickness.

The rate of sickness is known to follow a U curve—that is, the sickness rate is high in people who get too little sleep and in people who get too much sleep.

Sleeping 8.5 hrs. could be a little worse than sleeping 5 hrs.

Many diseases such as depression, obesity, and heart disease have been associated with these sleep patterns.

Amount of sleep required during intensive training periods:

Research conducted by Cheri Mah (Stanford Sleep Disorders Clinic and Research Laboratory) has revealed that increased amounts of sleep can play a huge role during intensive training periods.

It's been found that increased sleep improves sports performance for all types of athletes during the competitive season.

According to the study published by the Cheri Mah in 2009, the Stanford University women's tennis team improved their sprint time, accuracy of tennis shots, and overall performance when they increased their sleep time to ten hours per night and maintained it for a period of five weeks.

The athletes on the Stanford men's and women's swim teams and men's basketball team also reported better mood, better satisfaction, and alertness after extra sleep. Sleep debt is known to have a negative impact on sports performance, particularly for collegiate and professional athletes.

How is sleep linked to sports performance?

Growth hormone is released during sleep. Growth hormone is responsible for muscle growth, muscle repair, fat burning, bone growth, and recovery.

Sleep deprivation can directly affect these functions.

However, the good news is that the effects of sleep deprivation show up only after a few nights of poor sleep. A poor night of sleep due to nervousness just before the competition is not likely to hurt the athlete's performance.

Sleep architecture: Stages of sleep:

Sleep can be divided into two broad types: rapid eye movement (REM) and non-rapid eye movement (NREM) sleep.

NREM sleep can be further divided into in NREM stage 1, NREM stage 2, and NREM stage 3.

Sleep usually occurs in cycles of REM and NREM; usually four to five cycles can be seen per night. The normal order of sleep is N1 → N2 → N3 → N2 → REM (repeated four to five times per night).

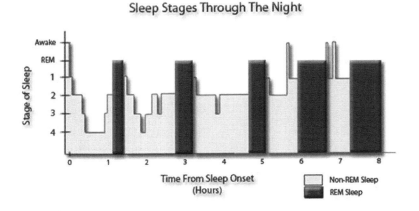

Sleep Stages Through The Night

Description of stages of sleep:

NREM stage 1:

During this stage, the person transitions from wakefulness to sleep. The brain activity transitions from alpha waves, which have a frequency of 8 to 13 Hz, to theta waves, which have a frequency of 4 to 7 Hz. The person usually appears to be drowsy during this stage, the muscles are usually active, and there is slow eye movement.

One can be awakened without difficulty; however, if aroused from this stage of sleep, one may feel as if one has not slept. Stage 1 may last for five to ten minutes. Many may notice the feeling of falling during this stage of sleep, which may cause a sudden muscle contraction (called hypnic myoclonia).

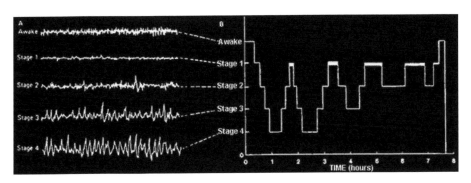

NREM stage 2:

In this stage the person slips deeper into sleep becomes harder to wake. This stage of sleep is characterized by theta brain activity. Sleep spindles and K complex also interrupt brain activity. The sleep spindles range from 11 to 16 Hz. During this stage the muscular activity decreases, and the conscious awareness of the surroundings diminishes. This stage takes up nearly 45 to 55 percent of the total sleep in adults.

This is a period of light sleep during which polysomnographic readings show intermittent peaks and valleys, or positive and negative waves. These waves indicate spontaneous periods of muscle tone mixed with periods of muscle relaxation. The heart rate slows and the body temperature decreases. At this point, the body enters deep sleep.

NREM stage 3:

This stage of sleep is formally divided into stages 3 and 4 (NREM 3 and 4). This stage is known as slow wave sleep or deep sleep. This stage of sleep is characterized by delta activity and high amplitude brainwaves (<3.5 Hz). During this stage the person is less responsive and reactive to the environment. This stage is notorious for night terrors, sleepwalking, and nocturnal enuresis.

During the deep stages of NREM sleep, the body repairs and regenerates tissues, builds bone and muscle, and appears to strengthen the immune system. As you get older, you sleep more lightly and get less deep sleep. Aging is also associated with shorter time spans of sleep, although studies show that the amount of sleep needed doesn't appear to diminish with age.

REM:

After the NREM stages of sleep, the subject enters the REM stage. The average adult reaches the REM sleep approximately every ninety minutes during sleep. This state of sleep is facilitated by acetylcholine secretion and inhibited by serotonin-secreting neurons. The subject also enters a stage of vivid dreaming.

The oxygen consumption during this stage is higher than when the sleeper is awake. During this stage of sleep, the muscles of the subject are paralyzed; this is also an evolutionary adaptation, so that the person does not physically move and react to his/her dreams.

How physiologic processes are linked to sleep and rest:

Our body follows a daily circadian rhythm to regulate physiologic processes in the body. Our circadian rhythms are generated and maintained by a structure in the brain known as the hypothalamus. The hypothalamus (suprachiasmatic nuclei) is responsible for our sleep-wake function and activity.

Circadian rhythms have a profound influence on hormonal regulation. The amount of growth hormone produced by the endocrine system is influenced directly by the circadian rhythm.

Studies published by Winget and Holly [1] confirm that these rhythms have the power to influence cognitive and physical performance of athletes. Many athletes report that their peak performance occurs during the afternoon period.

Any disruption in regular circadian rhythm cycle can prove to be a disadvantage to the athlete. Studies conducted by the Stanford University sleep disorders clinic showed that such minor alterations and disturbances in circadian rhythm can push back performance and thereby offer a substantial advantage to the opponent team in competitive situations.

Strategies and recommendations to promote better sleep in athletes:

1. Avoid intake of stimulants after 3:00 p.m.:

How can caffeine affects sports recovery and sleep?

In an effort to keep pace with the increasing demands of sport, many athletes try to use stimulants such as coffee and caffeine-based revitalizing drinks.

Caffeine is a mild stimulant; it's found in the stems, seeds, leaves, and roots of more than sixty-five plant species.

Caffeine stimulates the brain wave activity in tired people and arouses the mind. This is the most desired response for people who are sleep deprived.

Caffeine is also known to improve sports performance in athletes over the short term. A study conducted by Graham et al. (1998) revealed that athletes who consumed caffeine pills performed more efficiently than those who received the placebo.

The downside of caffeine:

Caffeine stimulates production of cortisol and pressurizes the adrenal glands to produce more stimulant hormones; it arouses many physiological responses, including the survival mechanism known as the flight-or-fight response. Caffeine stimulates the central nervous system and has a direct influence on the activity levels of the medulla and cortex; it even has the ability to reach the spinal cord when consumed in larger doses.

When caffeine consumption becomes a regular habit, it can worsen symptoms of adrenal fatigue and cause symptoms of burnout in the athlete. It can lead to easy fatigue, irritability, and cause a poor quality of mood during the day. Caffeine can also cause an increase in skeletal muscle tension and heart rate; it can also lead to heartburn, loss of focus, and fatigue.

Caffeine has a direct effect on the detrusor muscles of the bladder; this increases the urgency and frequency of urination, and this can lead to issues such as dehydration, muscle tightness, and muscle cramping in athletes.

Increased consumption of caffeine also causes a disturbance in sleep rhythms by producing increased levels of cortisol.

The International Olympic Committee (IOC) currently lists caffeine as a banned substance. It may be hard to believe that a substance such as caffeine, which is consumed by more than 75 percent of Americans every day, is placed in a category that includes harmful drugs such as steroids and cocaine. The IOC perceives a urinary test above 12mg/liter (eight cups of coffee) as a deliberate attempt by an athlete to gain an advantage over the competition.

Solution: Moderation is the key; consuming more than two cups of coffee can cause arousal of autonomic nervous system. Consuming coffee after 3:00 p.m. can influence the sleep rhythm during the night; hence, limiting coffee consumption to less than one or two cups per day and avoiding coffee intake after 3:00 p.m. can decrease stress and anxiety throughout the day in addition to facilitating healthy sleep rhythm during the night.

2. Avoid sports drinks that contain active stimulants:
Avoid drinks that contain yohimbe, geranium, guarana, methylsynephrine, citrus aurantium, ma-huang extract, or kola-nut extract.

Effect of stimulants on the body:

Even though the athlete may not intend to consume these stimulants, these may be passed around unwittingly in the training circuits by well meaning co-athletes and sports fans.

Sports stimulants push the adrenal glands to produce stimulatory hormones; they can change the circadian rhythm and cause the athlete to feel awake during the training session; however, it can affect the recovery period of athletes after training.

Sports drinks and stimulants that can affect the circadian rhythm and athlete recovery:

1) *Guarana* is a natural source of caffeine; it increases the risk for dehydration without any known benefit to the athlete or anyone else.

2) *Gotu kola* is another caffeine-like product with no known medical benefits. This too can increase the risk of dehydration.

3) *Caffeine* is a stimulant that increases the risk of dehydration and has limited benefit to athletes.

4) *Cocoa* or *Koka* may be indicated by a chocolate flavor; cocoa is another source of a caffeine-like stimulant that should be avoided in athletes.

5) *Methylsynephrine*, also known as oxilofrine, is a prohibited stimulant, but it's found in a few sports drinks.

6) *Citrus aurantium* is a source of synephrine and has stimulant properties.

7) *Ma huang* is a natural source of ephedra; it is a prohibited stimulant but still continues to exist in many sports drinks.

Methylhexaneamine	Geranium (extract, stems, or oil), geranamine, "geranium surge," and other made-up names; 1,3-Dimethylamyline, dimethylpentylamine
Octopamine	ß,4-Dihydroxyphenethylamine; p-Hydroxymandelamine; ND-50; Noroxedrine; p-Norsynephrine
Oxilofrine	Methylsynephrine
Phenpromethylamine	Fenprometamina, phenpromethamine, phenpromethaminum, phenylpropylmethylamine, "Benzedrine"

3. Avoid alcohol three hours before bedtime to avoid disturbed sleep patterns:

Alcohol consumption is known to cause sleep disruption and sleep disorders; long-term consumption of alcohol affects the time required to fall asleep (sleep latency) and alters the total sleep time.

When a person first consumes alcohol, it creates an initial stimulating effect; however, alcohol consumed one hour prior to bedtime is known to disrupt the second half of sleep. The second half of sleep is then marked by the improper quality of sleep, regular awakening from dreams, and difficulty going back to sleep. This disruption of sleep can lead to daytime tiredness and fatigue.

The sleep-inducing quality of alcohol decreases if the subject continues to use alcohol over a long period of time.

Studies [2] have also shown that moderate consumption of alcohol (one to two ounces spirit) six hours prior to sleep can cause sleep disruption during the second half of sleep. Even though the dose of alcohol consumed six hours prior to sleep is eliminated from the bloodstream, it continues to have a long-lasting effect on the quality of sleep.

4. Avoid large meals before bed:

Acid reflux: Eating large meals prior to bedtime can provoke an acid reflux in the stomach, which can lead to stomach irritation, discomfort, and low quality of sleep. For this reason it is best to avoid large meals two to three hours prior to bedtime.

Sleeplessness: Eating large meals fires up the metabolism, which makes it all the more difficult to fall asleep or maintain a high quality of sleep.

Weight gain: Research studies [3] have demonstrated a direct link between weight gain and heavy eating before bedtime. This partly happens because most of the calories obtained from the heavy meal are not utilized during sleep.

Snacks recommended for better quality of sleep:

New research [5] into sleep metabolism shows that two metabolic hormones, leptin and ghrelin, which were discovered during the last decade, could play a major role in the quality of sleep. Leptin is responsible for a feeling of satiety, whereas ghrelin stimulates hunger.

Researchers suggest that consumption of a small meal prior to bedtime produces enough leptin to suppress the secretion of ghrelin, so we'll sleep throughout the night without any feelings of hunger.

Snacks that contain tryptophan (amino acid) can act as great precursors to sleep, because tryptophan helps in production of serotonin.

The ideal snack before bedtime would be a combination of tryptophan (amino acids) and carbohydrate. This combination works well because all amino acids compete for transport into the brain; when carbohydrates are added to a meal, they trigger the release of insulin, which helps in the absorption of competing amino acids into the muscle tissue while leaving behind tryptophan, which can be readily transported to the brain.

Ideal size of bedtime snack: A snack containing 200–250 calories [4] should be adequate for the athlete to get through the night without any episodes of hypoglycemia.

Suggested bedtime snack:

- Low-fat granola bar

- One cup healthy cereal mixed with skim milk* (occasionally)

- Scoop of vanilla or strawberry low-fat ice cream

- Flavored non-fat yogurt topped with two to three tablespoons of low-fat cereal

- Low-fat popcorn sprinkled with Parmesan cheese

- A glass of milk* (occasionally)

- Handful of almonds

- Apple with peanut butter

- Casein protein shake made with water (approximately 200 calories).

What to avoid:

Avoid spicy foods, fried foods, heavy sugars, soda, red meat, and oatmeal.

*Milk contains high levels of calcium, which can reduce zinc and magnesium absorption; deficiency of zinc and magnesium can be very detrimental to athletic performance, and for this reason it is better to use milk only occasionally as a bedtime snack.

5. Consume foods that have natural relaxants:
Magnesium is regarded as one of the most powerful natural relaxants available.

According to the *Journal of Intensive Care Medicine*, [6] the deficiency of magnesium causes a long list of diseases.

Magnesium deficiency has been linked to higher levels of C-reactive protein and inflammation the body. High training volumes and sleep deprivation can lead to depleted magnesium levels that in turn cause restless leg syndrome: periodic limb movement during sleep.

Eating food rich in magnesium and consuming magnesium supplements can help avoid many diseases [7] and improve rates of recovery in athletes. Magnesium is widely regarded as an antidote to stress; it's known to improve the quality of your sleep.

The recommended daily allowance (RDA) for magnesium is 300 mg per day.

Sources of magnesium:
Kelp, wheat bran, peas, lentils, wheat germ, almonds, cashews, buckwheat, brazil nuts, dulse, filberts, millet, pecans, walnuts, rye, tofu, soy beans, brown rice, figs, dates, collard greens, shrimp, avocado, parsley, beans, barley, dandelion greens, and garlic

Foods that drain magnesium from the body are coffee, colas, salt, sugar, and alcohol.

6. Use light to your advantage:

Certain hormones, such as melatonin, in our body are influenced by exposure to light.

Light therapy: If an athlete suffers from sleep deprivation, it is especially useful to expose the athlete to full-spectrum lights (10,000 lux fluorescent bulbs) for a period of fifteen to thirty minutes between 7.30 and 8:00 a.m.

It's been found that such exposure to full-spectrum light triggers the nighttime release of melatonin; this helps the person fall asleep earlier and stay asleep longer. These full-spectrum light boxes cost between $100 and $150 and can be easily purchased on websites such as eBay and Amazon.com.

7. Create a nighttime sleep ritual:

A night of proper sleep can serve as a great source of energy. According to Dr. Epstein, co-author of *The Harvard Medical School Guide to a Good Night's Sleep*, creating a pre-sleep ritual trains our body to expect what's coming.

If we make a habit of reading prior to bedtime, then the body immediately starts associating reading with bedtime. Certain conditions ensure optimal sleep; let's explore the dos and don'ts for good sleep in the following section.

a) *Identify the time to wind down:* To do this first, identify the ideal time you'd like to wake up in the morning. Next count backward by about seven hours and designate a separate fifteen-minute period to start your wind-down process and sleep ritual. Try adding one hour of sleep and check if it improves how you feel and perform throughout the day.

b) *Create a cozy sleeping environment:* A 2001 German study on sleep revealed that dim lighting, mildly cold temperature, and a medium-firm pillow improved the quality of sleep considerably.

A non-allergenic foam pillow with a dust-mite-blocking protector can significantly reduce the amount of allergies that hinder proper breathing during sleep.

The environment may change depending on where you live; some areas of the country are colder and the homes become very dry due to the type of heating systems. It is imperative that you use a humidifier, so that your first line of defense—a moist nasal and throat passage—is maintained. If the nasal tissues become dry, they are more susceptible to transmission of bacteria and viruses.

c) *Use the bathroom:* A hot (or cold) bath is known to help calm down the brain activity.

d) *Block blue light spectrum:* Reduce the amount of stimuli you get from electronic devices such as computer and TV during the evening. Studies have revealed that the blue spectrum light emitted by computers, digital clocks, DVD player readouts, televisions, and other digital devices can harm the body's natural biorhythm, especially late at night. For this reason it is advisable to switch off or cover all the light emitted by the digital devices and keep your room pitch dark at night.

e) *Avoid staying awake in bed:* Best sleep practices developed by Harvard University suggest that if you don't fall asleep within twenty minutes of going to bed, you should get up and move around until you feel sleepy. Do not indulge in stimulating activities such as watching TV, eating, planning, or problem-solving; instead try reading a book.

Reading a fiction book or having someone reading to you can help you disconnect from the real world and pressures and help you relax better. Fifteen to twenty minutes of reading is found to promote relaxation.

If reading a book does not appeal to you, then you may try listening to calming music, stretching, or doing relaxation exercises.

You can also add biofeedback devices or apps such as "stress ensure"—these are instruments to lower stress, and they will be discussed in the following chapters.

f) *Supplements that promote good sleep:*

Melatonin has a direct influence on the sleep cycle. Levels of melatonin increase just before you fall asleep and decline throughout the sleep period. Melatonin can be very helpful in resetting the sleep rhythm. Melatonin supplementation can especially prove useful to athletes who undertake a hectic travel schedule across different time zones.

The recommended dosage of melatonin for resetting the sleep rhythm is 1–3 mg two hours before sleep time. It is important to remember that melatonin is not a sleeping pill; instead, it helps only in resetting the sleep rhythm.

Valerian is often known as the herbal sleeping pill. Valerian is more powerful than chamomile when it comes to sedative powers. Valerian should be avoided before performing heavy tasks and before driving. The recommended dose is 400 to 600 mg two hours before bedtime.

Anti-stress pill L-theanine: Theanine is an amino acid with calming properties. Theanine helps reduce tension and alleviates stress. Suntheanine 200 mg (a special type of theanine) is recommended, along with a B-complex vitamin, during the evening time for stress release. The recommended brand is NOW Foods.

Tylenol PM is a useful aid to relieve pain fast and ensure sleep. It provides relief from headaches, minor aches, and sleeplessness.

Ambien, or zolpidem, is used to treat insomnia (difficulty falling asleep or staying asleep). Zolpidem belongs to a class of medications called sedative-hypnotics. It works by slowing activity in the brain and promotes sleep.

Zolpidem (Ambien) side effects:

Ambien can cause side effects; it has been related to several allergic reactions. You should stop intake of zolpidem and get medical treatment immediately if you notice any signs of allergy, which include difficulty breathing, and swelling of your face, lips, tongue, or throat.

Call your doctor immediately if you notice any of these serious side effects:

- Pain in the chest, fast or irregular heartbeat, feeling short of breath

- Trouble breathing or swallowing

- Feeling like you might pass out

Other less serious side effects of zolpidem may include the following:

- Daytime drowsiness, dizziness, or weakness; feeling "drugged" or light-headed

- Tired feeling; loss of coordination

- Dry mouth; nose or throat irritation

- Nausea, constipation, diarrhea, or upset stomach

- Stuffy nose; sore throat

- Headache; muscle pain

Tryptophan is an essential amino acid; it cannot be produced by our body and hence must be consumed through our diet.

Tryptophan helps in the production of serotonin and niacin; it was used as a sleep aid for many years, until it was banned due to outbreak of eosinophilia myalgia syndrome caused by impurities present in L-tryptophan supplied by a Japanese manufacturer and due to the use of large dosages.

Tryptophan was later brought back in 2005 at a very low dose.

Warm milk as sleep aid?

Milk protein contains alpha-lactalbumin, which is a natural protein source with the highest tryptophan content relative to other large neutral amino acids; it is found in human breast milk and cow's milk.

However, the principle protein in cow's milk is beta-lactoglobulin, a low-tryptophan protein that is not found in human milk. So milk is not an ideal bedtime drink; in addition, the high calcium levels in milk can reduce zinc and magnesium uptake, which are both very important for growth and recovery.

Reserve your bed for only sleep and intimacy. Do not use your bed to watch TV, or do computer work or paperwork; sleep programs developed by the Harvard medical school advise that the bed be used only for sleep and intimacy.

Avoid watching TV until you fall asleep.

Avoid reading heavy-action novels prior to sleep, since they may cause you to ignore your sleep.

Avoid watching movies after 10:00 p.m., since watching them can prolong the time it takes to wind down and get into a comfortable sleep mood.

Switch off all your media at a specific time; if you have computer work to be done late at night, try shifting it to early morning.

Beware of the seven sleep stealers:
The seven major sleep stealers are as follows:

- Health issues

- Anxiety and stress

- Disruptive bedroom environment

- Inconsistent sleep schedule

- Stimulating nighttime activities

- Poor sleep diet

- Bedmates: kids and pets

g) *The psychology behind sleep:*
Practice mind exercises for worry distraction. The brain can usually engage in only one activity at a time. If you have written down your worries and find that your worries still don't go away, then you can try using one of the following games for worry distraction:

- Practice turning off your thoughts.

- Try to think of fruits that start with a particular alphabet: start with *A* and move up to *Z*.

- Try simple multiplication, division, and addition in your head; this forces your brain to move away from worrying, stressful thoughts and focus your mind on plain, unemotional thoughts.

- Imagine a certain object that relaxes you and try to vividly imagine what you would smell, hear, touch, and feel when you hold or touch such an object.

- Counting down from 30 to 1; inhalation on 30 and exhalation on 29; when your mind wanders, start again.

Maintain a journal. Silberman, author of *The Insomnia Workbook: A Comprehensive Guide to Getting the Sleep You Need*, talks about the effect of writing down your worries for ten to fifteen minutes a day.

Listing your worries and concerns for ten to fifteen minutes and then writing a proposed plan of action can reduce the amount of stress and worries. She suggests asking the question, "What are the things that come to my mind when I'm lying in bed at night?"

Silberman advices that you stay away from the worry book prior to sleep, just to allow some separation from thoughts that concern you; if a worrying thought comes up right before bed or during bedtime, you can mentally check it off, and either say to yourself "I've dealt with that," or "I'm dealing with it."

Practice exercises for muscle relaxation. The following technique is advised by the Benson- Henry Institute for Mind-Body Medicine; this technique has produced many beneficial results and is approved by the Harvard Medical School.

ELICITATION OF THE RELAXATION RESPONSE

Elicitation of the relaxation response is actually quite easy. There are two essential steps:

1) Repetition of a word, sound, phrase, prayer, or muscular activity

2) Passive disregard of everyday thoughts that inevitably come to mind and the return to your repetition

The following is the generic technique taught at the Benson-Henry Institute:

1) Pick a focus word, short phrase, or prayer that is firmly rooted in your belief system, such as *one, peace, The Lord is my shepherd, Hail Mary full of grace,* or *shalom.*

2) Sit quietly in a comfortable position.

3) Close your eyes.

4) Relax your muscles, progressing from your feet to your calves, thighs, abdomen, shoulders, head, and neck.

5) Breathe slowly and naturally, and, as you do, say your focus word, sound, phrase, or prayer silently to yourself as you exhale.

6) Assume a passive attitude. Don't worry about how well you're doing. When other thoughts come to mind, simply say to yourself, "Oh well," and gently return to your repetition.

7) Continue for ten to twenty minutes.

8) Do not stand immediately. Continue sitting quietly for a minute or so, allowing other thoughts to return. Then open your eyes, and sit for another minute before rising.

9) Practice the technique once or twice daily. Good times to do so are before breakfast and before dinner.

Regular elicitation of the relaxation response has been scientifically proven to be an effective treatment for a wide range of stress-related disorders. In fact, to the extent that any disease is caused or made worse by stress, the relaxation response can help.

Techniques for evoking the relaxation response just before going to sleep:

Observation meditation:

Total time required: Three minutes:

A more intense form of meditation is to sit and note what is happening. Thoughts will arise and subside, and your task is to let them pass through your mind.

It's a form of *mindfulness*, which is a deliberate sort of awareness, whereby the meditator closes off the external world, to the best of his or her ability, and becomes more consciously aware of the patterns of thoughts.

How is it helpful?

This technique is an excellent stress-reliever. It helps us slow down, disengage from the chaos of the day, and become one with our own mind. Over time it can result in a faster mind, sharp problem-solving skills, and a more holistic manner of perception.

For all that, it's quite easy!

The steps:

1) Begin by getting relaxed. Wear loose, non-restrictive clothing, and sit yourself in a comfortable position. Over time you'll probably find you can meditate—using this technique or any other—in a variety of postures, from standing to lying down.

It's best to start this technique, though, in a comfortable sitting position, back straight, feet flat on the floor, and arms at your sides or in your lap.

2) Close your eyes, or leave them open—whichever is most comfortable for you.

3) Just sit and relax, and—*breathe*. Breathe deeply, in and out. Draw the air in fully, hold for just a second, then let it fully out.

4) As you're doing so, focus your attention—fully, completely—on your breath. To the highest degree you can, think about nothing except the air moving in and moving out.

5) Now of course, your attention will wander. It's inevitable, because that's what our minds do. But *mindfulness* gives us the ability, the understanding, to be consciously aware of that. You will *know* when your attention has shifted away from the slow, steady rhythm of your breathing.

And when it does, just say to yourself, "I'm thinking." Just make note of the shift in attention, and steer your focus back to your breathing.

6) You don't want to get stressed about the shifting attention, and you don't want to get angry with yourself when your attention shifts. If you are a beginner your attention will most certainly shift. For an experienced meditator the attention seldom shifts and they enjoy a deep state of awareness.

At this point I'd like to remind you that mindfulness is neutral. It's not about making judgments over your ability, or inability, to hold focus. It's about watching that process of wandering attention, learning from it, training it, and improving it over time.

7) By the same token, it's not unusual for strange thoughts, even disturbing thoughts, to arise when we're mindfully Being the Watcher. That's OK. Once again, just relax, and come back to your breathing. Just notice the thought, make note of it, and tell yourself, "This is just a thought. It isn't me." Let it go, and guide your focus back to slow, steady breathing. Relax. Breathe in; breathe out.

8) Do this exercise for about three minutes during your first session. Let your breathing return to its original, carefree state—to its original natural rhythm, in other words.

Continue this exercise for the next three minutes.

9) After three minutes have passed, open your eyes.

Spend some time reflecting on what your thoughts were like and where they took you.

Imagine how relaxed you would feel if you trained your mind to practice mindfulness for ten minutes every day, or for a half hour, or even an hour. Just spend some time picturing where your mind might have gone and what it would have been like watching that.

How long and how often it should be done:

Do this exercise for three minutes per session prior to sleep, up to three times a week in the beginning. Gradually work your way up to five to seven sessions per week.

After you feel comfortable with the exercise, you can slowly work your way up to ten-minute and twenty-minute sessions. You can even choose to do extended, one-hour sessions on weekends and holidays.

What results can you expect?

As you do this exercise, you will realize that your mind becomes calmer, and you'll start feeling more comfortable in your own skin. You will notice that your body feels relaxed, along with your mind, and getting through a long workday will seem a lot easier.

Here's an additional tip: as you get accustomed to the exercise, cultivate a tendency for mindfulness—an ability to stop at any time, in any situation, and fully experience your inner and outer environment. It is perhaps the best way to be "in the moment," and you'll find it'll give you a clearer mind and a greater appreciation for life than you ever thought possible.

Other recommended relaxation routines include the following:

- Imagery: guided imagery via audio tape or self-guided imagery and visualization

- Repetitive prayer

- Mindfulness meditation

- Repetitive physical exercises

- Mindful Breathing: practicing relaxed diaphragmatic breathing. Deep mindful breathing is linked to reduced levels of oxidative stress, decreased cortisol, and increased levels of melatonin (Martarelli et al. 2009 Italian study)

You may want to try more than one technique to find the one that suits you best.

If you are a trainer, you may advise the athlete to practice all the above-mentioned tips and try to incorporate the practices into his/her daily schedule in a stepwise manner. In order to further monitor sleep complaints, you can ask the athlete to maintain a sleep diary for at least two months and study the impact of each of the above-mentioned tips. A review of the sleep diary every one to two months can bring about drastic changes in sleep patterns and quality of relaxation.

Benefits of meditation and relaxation:

- Increased energy levels

- Decreased stress levels

- Decrease in oxidative stress

- Increased focus

- Increased positive self-image

- Increase in awareness of state

The effective use of napping:

In order to understand how naps can be used effectively throughout the day to promote relaxation and recovery, we need to understand the physiology of sleep.

Even though a forty-five-minute nap may appear to be a better idea than a twenty-minute nap, the reality is somewhat different.

Our sleep goes through five stages.

Sleep stage 1 typically lasts for about ten minutes, and stage 2 lasts for another ten minutes. If your nap takes you from stage 1 sleep (just drifting off) to stage 2 (brain activity slows), you will wake up feeling energized and more alert.

If your nap takes you into stages 3 and 4 (deep sleep), you will not wake easily and will feel groggy and tired.

How you feel upon waking up really depends on the stage of sleep that you've woken up from. Here's a brief explanation of how you may feel after waking from different stages of sleep.

Short nap: A person will enter into NREM2 after twenty minutes of sleep; if the athlete is woken up at twenty minutes of sleep, this person will still wake up without feeling groggy.

Research on pilots shows that a twenty-six-minute "NASA" nap in flight (while the plane is manned by a copilot) enhanced performance by 34 percent and overall alertness by 54 percent.

Impact on memory: a 2008 study in Düsseldorf showed that the onset of sleep may trigger active memory processes that remain effective even if sleep is limited to only a few minutes.

Long nap: One-and-a-half to two hours of sleep—this will take you through a full sleep cycle, and you will wake up feeling refreshed.

Bad nap: When athletes sleep for forty-five minutes, it's very likely that they have entered NREM3 (deep sleep); if they are woken up at such a stage, then they feel groggy from the effects of sleep inertia.

What is the best time to take a nap?

The best time to take a nap is between one and three in the afternoon; this is because the levels of melatonin rise during that time, which in turn creates a drop in energy level.

Animal behavior studies reveal that many mammals sleep for short periods throughout the day. Humans are the only mammals to have consolidated their sleep habit into one long period; however, our bodies are programmed for two periods of intense sleepiness: in the early morning, from about two to four, and in the afternoon between one and three o'clock, due to melatonin modulation.

Tips to nap better:

- Using a set of earplugs and eye covers can help you nap more effectively.

- Nap for twenty minutes.

- Nap between one and three in the afternoon.

- Try to avoid taking a nap within three hours of bedtime, as this may delay your nighttime sleep.

The caffeine nap: Research studies in Japan[8] have shown that subjects who try to nap for ten to twenty minutes after consuming a cup of coffee report feeling more refreshed after waking up; the extra energy from the coffee and the nap helped them feel more alert and awake after a short nap.

Caffeine requires twenty or thirty minutes to take effect, so it will kick in just as you're waking. A research study revealed that the caffeine nap was more effective in terms of increased productivity and decreased levels of sleepiness when compared with subjects who took only a nap and washed their face, or took a nap and were exposed to bright working lights.

Sleep inertia: Forty years ago, the US Air Force and NASA tested the ability of pilots sleeping in the cockpit to wake up and immediately take flight. Most pilots made many errors; it was later discovered that extreme grogginess occurs when a person wakes up from deep sleep.

They then coined the term *sleep inertia*. Most sleep aids find a moment when you are not in deep sleep and wake you with an alarm; this makes the process somewhat easier.

Sleep tools:

- <u>Sleep Cycle</u>: iPhone app, which be found at the online iTunes store ($0.99)

  How it works: An intelligent alarm clock analyzes your sleep and wakes you in the lightest sleep phase—the natural way to wake up feeling rested and relaxed. Sleep Cycle monitors your movement during sleep using the extremely sensitive accelerometer in your iPhone. Sleep Cycle then finds the optimal time to wake you up during a thirty-minute window that ends at your set alarm time.

- <u>Stress Doctor</u>: iPhone app, which can be found at the online iTunes store

  How it works: It reduces your stress by using a 100 percent natural biofeedback technique based on heart rate detection with your iPhone's camera.

- <u>Stress Check</u>: iPhone app, which can be found at the online iTunes store

  How it works: Stress Check is the most innovative iPhone tool available for quantifying your level of psychological or physical stress. By measuring your heart rate through the camera and light features on your iPhone, Stress Check can estimate your level of stress in real time. The app requires you to place your index finger on your iPhone camera lens, after which it starts measuring your heart rate and stress levels.

- Zeo

How it works: The Zeo is a sleep-monitoring device that keeps track of the amount of time spent in each stage of sleep and then gives it a score. It uses a headband to help you track your sleep patterns and estimates how much restorative REM and deep sleep you actually get; the information is then sent to your smartphone along with recommendations, so you can better manage your health and overall wellness.

Fitbit Device:

The Fitbit Ultra monitors your all-day activity to provide you with real-time feedback on steps, distance, calories burned, and stairs climbed to encourage you to walk more and be more active. It wirelessly uploads your data to Fitbit.com so you can gain deeper insight into your daily or monthly fitness and sleep levels with free online graphs and charts. On Fitbit.com, you can earn fitness badges, connect with friends to share and compete on fitness goals, or join the Fitbit community for advice and encouragement.

Benefits of Fitbit:

- Tracks steps, distance, calories burned, and stairs climbed, with a 3D accelerometer and altimeter

- Measures how long and how well you sleep

- Wirelessly uploads data to Fitbit.com

- View charts and graphs for daily and monthly progress online or with the free

- iPhone app

- Log food and workouts online and with iPhone app

- Access Food Goal, a weight management tools that dynamically changes targets based on daily activities

- Small, discreet design fits into a pocket or clips to a belt or bra

For more information go to http://www.fitbit.com/home

Jawbone UP:

Jawbone UP is a system that takes a holistic approach to a healthy lifestyle. The wristband tracks your movement and sleep in the background. The app displays your data, lets you add things such as meals and mood, and delivers insights that keep you moving forward.

https://jawbone.com/up

- StressEraser: StressEraser is an FDA-regulated, portable biofeedback device that helps you learn to activate your body's natural relaxation response in minutes—without the use of medication.

How it works: From beat to beat, your heart rate naturally increases and decreases in a cycle, known as HRV, or heart rate variability. Using a harmless infrared sensor, the StressEraser measures HRV from the pulse in your fingertip. It then uses simple symbols—squares and triangles—to cue your breathing with your heart rate cycle, thereby reducing stress.

References:

(1)   Winget and Holly. Circadian rhythms and performance. *Med Sci Sports Exercise Journal.*

(2)   Landolt, H. P., et al. Late-afternoon ethanol intake affects nocturnal sleep and the sleep EEG in middle-aged men. *J Clin Psychopharmacol* 16(6):428–436, 1996.

(2)   Vitiello, M. V. Sleep, alcohol and alcohol abuse. *Addict Biol* (2): 151–158, 1997.

(3)   Arble, D. Mouse-model study conducted by Northwestern University, 2009.

(4)   http://today.msnbc.msn.com/id/23003124/ns/today-today_health/t/eat-your-way-good-nights-sleep/#.UO1AMuRJ4wI

(5)   http://www.webmd.com/sleep-disorders/features/trouble-sleeping-some-bedtime-snacks-can-help-you-sleep

(6)   Tong, G.M. and R. K. Rude. Magnesium deficiency in critical illness. *J Intensive Care Med* 20 (1):3–17, 2005. Review.

(7)   Johnson, S. The multifaceted and widespread pathology of magnesium deficiency. *Med Hypotheses* 56(2):163–70, 2001.

(8)   Hayashi, M., A. Masuda, and T. Hori. The alerting effects of caffeine, bright light and face washing after a short daytime nap. *Clin Neurophysiol.* 114(12):2268–78, 2003.

The Third Pillar of Recovery

Play

The Third Pillar of Recovery: Play

PLAY FORMS AN IMPORTANT PART OF RECOVERY AND performance; most human motivations are ultimately toward pleasure (play) and away from pain.

When an athlete chooses sport as a serious profession, it shifts from being a source of recreation and fun to being a source of livelihood, high expectations, and measure for self-worth.

Due to the professional pressures, it is very easy for the athlete to forget the importance of fun and play in day-to-day life. However, play cannot be ignored, because it can have a positive impact on life and produce a measurable improvement in performance.

Play can include any activity that fosters positive emotions and encourages people to connect better with their friends and family. It can include smiling and laughter, getting to know other people, learning about another person, engaging in a mutual interest, and more.

Play cannot be a forced activity; instead, it should encourage creativity and build the self-esteem of the group.

According to the National Institute, play is the gateway to vitality. By incorporating play and pleasure into daily life, the athlete tends to develop an optimistic look toward life; play also fosters healthy relationships, a better immune system, and a positive mental attitude.

Playful communication sets up the foundation for deeper and more rewarding relationships with friends and family; it also creates a sense of intimacy.

Let's look at some of the activities that can be considered as play:

1) Laughter.

2) Hobbies: Finding something outside of sport that is for pure fun and helps relieve stress.

3) Combining family and hobbies.

4) Turning family and friends into a source of support instead of stress, pressure, and entourage.

5) Play also means learning effective methods to shield yourself from the bad habits of friends and family and not let their bad habits affect you.

6) The athlete also needs to prevent exercise from turning into an obsession that can impact the athlete's career negatively.

1. Laughter:

What is laughter, really?

When we laugh heartily, changes occur in many parts of the body, even the arms, legs, and trunk muscles.

Science studies reveal that laughter is different from other emotional reactions in the brain; laughter activates all parts of the brain.

What we laugh in response to:

- Humor

- Enjoyment of novelty: for example, the sight of a beautiful landscape or unexpected surprise

- To show rapport: for example, while sharing a lighthearted sense of the world's ironies

- Sharing experiences: the enjoyment of mutual storytelling

- Sharing imagination: the capacity to openly divulge imagination and fantasies

Brain experiments reveal that almost all areas of the brain are activated by laughter; the following research findings are noteworthy:

- The key benefit of laughter is that it lights up all parts of the brain, whereas other types of emotional reactions are confined to only one part of the brain.

- The brain's large frontal lobe, which is involved in social emotional responses, becomes very active.

- The words and structure of the joke are analyzed by the left side of the cortex.

- The intellectual analysis required to "get" the joke is carried out by the right hemisphere of the cortex.

- Brainwave activity then spread to the sensory processing area of the occipital lobe (the area on the back of the head that contains the cells that process visual signals).

- The physical responses to the joke are evoked by the stimulation of the motor sections.

According to cultural anthropologist Mahadev Apte, "Laughter occurs when people are comfortable with one another, when they feel open and free. And the more laughter, the more bonding within the group."

As children we found almost everything funny; that's because as infants and children, we were constantly discovering the world around us. For kids, a lot of what goes on seems ridiculous and surprising and very often strikes them as funny; the same jokes would be brushed off by most adults as childish or ridiculous!

As we mature, both our physical bodies and mental outlooks grow and change; throughout our life we experience success and tragedy at much deeper levels, and the childish sense of wonder and curiosity is lost in most adults.

Benefits of laughter:

- Laughter relaxes the whole body. A good, hearty laugh relieves physical tension and stress, leaving your muscles relaxed for up to forty-five minutes after.

- Laughter boosts the immune system. Laughter decreases stress hormones and increases immune cells and infection-fighting antibodies, thus improving your resistance to disease.

  Research studies have proven that laughing stimulates the production of natural killer cells that destroy tumors and viruses; laughter is also known to increase the rate of production of Gamma-interferon (proteins that fight disease); T-cells, which are a major part of the immune response; and B-cells, which are responsible for the production of disease-destroying antibodies.

  The concentration of *salivary immunoglobulin A*, which defends against infectious organisms entering through the respiratory tract, is increased during laughter.

- Laughter triggers the release of endorphins, the body's natural feel-good chemicals. Endorphins promote an overall sense of well-being and can even temporarily relieve pain.

- Laughter protects the heart. Laughter improves the function of blood vessels and increases blood flow, which can help protect you against a heart attack and other cardiovascular problems.

- Laughter is cathartic: According to the American Association for Therapeutic Humor, most people store emotions such as anger, fear, and sadness instead of finding a creative outlet to these negative emotions. Laughter can prove to be very beneficial in such situations. A trip to the comedy club, watching funny movies, or having a good laugh with your friends and family can help release these negative emotions.

The whole concept of laughter therapy is based upon teaching people on how to laugh openly and use laughter to cope with difficult situations that aren't usually funny.

How to bring more laughter into your life

- Be funny every chance you get—as long as you are not putting anybody down!

- Figure out what makes people in your life laugh, and do it more often.

- Surround yourself with people who laugh.

- Read funny articles, books, and comic strips.

- Watch comedy movies and TV shows.

- Develop your own sense of humor. Read a book or two on how to be a better comic. Here's a good book by Melvin Helitzer: *Comedy Writing Secrets*.

2. Hobbies: Finding something outside of sport that is pure fun:

Very often it is easy for an athlete to get caught up between the responsibilities of family and career and have little energy or time left for relaxing hobbies such as crafts, music, or painting.

Much like meditation, active hobbies such as music, painting, and crafts can provide a total change of focus and shift in mood.

The key to enjoying these hobbies while performing well in your career and family is to incorporate a few minutes devoted to these activities every day; this allows you to reap the psychological rewards of engaging in hobbies.

Dr. S. Ausim Azizi, chairman of the department of neurology at Temple University's School of Medicine in Philadelphia, who studies brain activity and cell signaling, says that involving in a hobby activates a specific part of the brain called the nucleus accumbens, which affects how you feel about life. Not only that, an activity or craft that you enjoy can stimulate the brain's septal zone (the feel-good area) and make you feel happier.

According to Dr. Carol Kauffman, assistant professor at Harvard Medical School, whenever people are completely engaged in an activity that they enjoy doing, they lose sense of time and enter a special state of mind known as the flow state. Any activity that allows a person to become completely engaged helps improve creativity and induces the flow state, which comes with its own set of benefits. The brain produces feel-good chemicals such as norepinephrine, endorphins, and dopamine during this heightened state; these chemicals help you stay focused, energized, and interested in what you are doing.

Dr. Gabriela Corá, a psychiatrist at the Florida Neuroscience Center, says, "Making time for enjoyable activities stimulates parts of the brain associated with creative and positive thinking. You become emotionally and intellectually more motivated."

Having a hobby that is completely different from the athlete's career can help the athlete enjoy the activity without being financially concerned about the outcome.

When people depend only on their career to foster a healthy sense of self-esteem, it often fails to be a consistent source of satisfaction and fulfillment; on the other hand, relying on a hobby to act as a source of a quick getaway can replenish a person's energy and self-esteem.

Having a hobby helps you identify yourself in multiple roles—as a sports person, painter, cook, artist, and so on. It helps you become multidimensional and derive your sense of identity from multiple sources instead of just your career.

The added creativity and confidence generated from the hobby can also help athletes perform well in their careers. Hobbies can also help motivate a person just prior to a major event; for example, if an athlete is interested in classical music, listening to a great piece of classical music just prior to a major event can help pump up the athlete and reduce feelings of nervousness.

How to make time for a hobby in your life:

- Start by thinking how a hobby can help you relax on a personal level.

- Try to think of a hobby as a meaningful event instead of a time-consuming distraction.

- After you have decided on your mental attitude, you can move to the next step, which is scheduling an activity on your calendar.

- You may try to pick a time early in the morning, or in the evening, or during the weekend. Test and choose the time that works best for you.

Qualities to look for when you choose a hobby:

1) You should have a genuine interest in the hobby.

2) It should have the potential of being a long-term interest.

3) It should make you feel good/positive.

4) It should be affordable and not expensive over the long term.

5) Never enter a hobby with an attitude of getting or gaining something.

Combining family and hobbies:

Once in a while you may consider combining family and hobbies.

Schedule the "helping hour" every week: make time to be attentive to others. The helping hour is an hour you reserve each week to completely focus on your friends, family, and their needs. It's a way of physically being present for them and helping them out in person rather than just financially. You might also consider participating or helping them out in their hobbies.

The Fourth Pillar of Recovery

Nutrition

The Fourth Pillar of Recovery: Nutrition

FOOD AND ITS IMPORTANCE WITH PERFORMANCE ATHLETES IS no secret, and the amount of information available in this area continues to grow.

Nutrition is an important component for maintaining a healthy and fruitful career in sports. Healthy nutrition can supply the body with all the important nutrients, vitamins, and minerals; absence of these vital nutrients in the diet can make the athlete feel weak, sick, and tired.

A well-balanced and well-planned diet is the key to experiencing success in sports.

Everything that athletes consume can have a direct impact on their weight management, immune system, and recovery process.

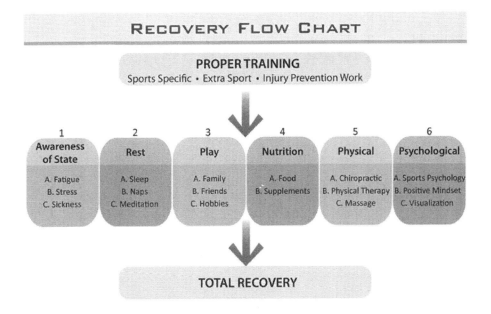

RECOVERY FLOW CHART

PROPER TRAINING
Sports Specific • Extra Sport • Injury Prevention Work

1 Awareness of State	2 Rest	3 Play	4 Nutrition	5 Physical	6 Psychological
A. Fatigue B. Stress C. Sickness	A. Sleep B. Naps C. Meditation	A. Family B. Friends C. Hobbies	A. Food B. Supplements	A. Chiropractic B. Physical Therapy C. Massage	A. Sports Psychology B. Positive Mindset C. Visualization

TOTAL RECOVERY

Exercise Feeding/Timing:

Exercise and feeding requirements are drastically different in serious athletes when compared to casual exercisers. Whenever an athlete undertakes strenuous physical activity, there is an excess amount of energy spent during the training that is well above the normal daily energy expenditure; the athlete also has increased requirements for specific types of nutrients such as carbohydrates.

Research studies [29b] have revealed that the energy expenditure among serious athletes is two to three times higher during exercise than for the sedentary individual. The energy is spent not only on training but also on recovery; it's estimated that nearly 40 percent of the total energy expenditure occurs during training (Danforth 1985) and the rest of the energy is consumed during recovery.

There are many factors that affect energy expenditure; these factors include body size, rate of muscular growth, muscular development, and recovery. The required amount of energy varies according to the athlete, and improper calculation can give rise to many methodological errors.

How often should you consume meals during the competition?

Research on eating patterns of various athletes:

- Tri-athletes who were surveyed reported an average of nine eating sessions daily.[40]

- Runners reported an average of five to six eating sessions daily. [41]

- Cyclists reported consuming an average of eight to ten meals daily. [42]

All the athletes reported that consuming a series of small meals and snacks throughout the day helped them maintain the required levels of energy while also reducing the gastric discomfort that may be caused by infrequent large meals.

Pre-exercise nutrition:

The main aim of pre-exercise nutrition is to:
1) Optimize the liver and muscle glycogen stores,

2) Avoid sudden increases in plasma insulin concentration (that can cause rebound hypoglycemia), and

3) Avoid stomach discomfort during exercise.

The pre-exercise period can be defined as a four-hour period prior to the event and can be divided into two stages that are metabolically significant: the two- to four-hour pre-exercise, and a thirty- to sixty-minute period pre-exercise. [43]

The two- to four-hour pre-exercise:
The type of meal required prior to the exercise greatly depends on the previous levels of recovery and carbohydrate intake.

Athletes who consume a carbohydrate rich diet for two to three days prior to the competition (carbohydrate loading) and reduce the exercise intensity will have an increased levels of glycogen, whereas the athletes that participate in strenuous exercise daily without any changes in diet prior to the event will enter the pre-exercise period with lower levels of muscle and liver glycogen stores.

It's been found that a carbohydrate-rich meal consumed four hours prior to the exercise greatly increases the muscle and liver glycogen content prior to exercise. [44] Research studies have also proven that a large amount of carbohydrates (around 300 g) consumed four hours prior to exercise improves the time taken to complete a fixed amount of work after prolonged, moderate-intensity cycling, compared to subjects who do not consume carbohydrates prior to the event. [45]

Similar results were reported when large meals were consumed three to four hours prior to moderate-intensity cycling. This improvement in performance is due to elevated levels of muscle glycogen.

The thirty- to sixty-minute period pre-exercise:

When compared to unfed athletes, the increased levels of plasma glucose and insulin in athletes who consumed carbohydrates thirty to sixty-minutes prior to exercise enjoyed an added advantage in performance.

However, it should be noted that certain individuals are susceptible to hyper-insulinemia associated with pre-exercise feeding, which may reduce the blood glucose level after the onset of exercise; however, this obstacle can be overcome by manipulating the timing of carbohydrate feeding or by choosing carbohydrates with a low glycemic index.

It should be noted that testing is the best judge of performance; therefore, an athlete must experiment with carbohydrate consumption and decide if it would provide the extra winning edge that she or he is looking for during the competition.

There are four major nutritional components that the athlete needs to pay attention to and experiment with when it comes to exercise feeding.

The four major nutritional components:

1) Water: to replace fluid lost as sweat and to aid the process of glycogen fixation

2) Electrolytes: to replenish minerals lost in sweat

3) Carbohydrates: to replenish muscle glycogen, the body's fuel

4) Protein: to repair and regenerate muscle fibers damaged during exercise; to promote muscle growth and adaptation

Water:

Water has one of the most powerful effects on human physiology; of all the factors that can reduce performance, water plays the largest role. Every organ in the body consists of more than 50 percent water.

Blood plasma is 92 percent water, and therefore, dehydration reduces the volume of blood in the body, which makes the cardiorespiratory system work harder to pump the blood around the body and deliver sufficient oxygen to the working muscles.

Water is our body's most essential fuel. Staying well hydrated is the key to a successful performance, and it is an important part of recovery.

Many studies have demonstrated that even a 1 percent (body weight) loss of water can reduce the performance in both power sports and endurance sports; it can lead to a state of dehydration and reduced aerobic endurance.

As the percentage of dehydration continues to rise, the athlete risks suffering more side effects. A 3 percent (body weight) loss of water can significantly reduce muscle endurance.

A 4 percent (body weight) loss of water can reduce muscle strength, decrease fine motor skills, produce heat cramps, and lead to other metabolic problems.

The major problem with dehydration is that it cannot be felt until the water loss reaches at least 2 percent of the body weight; at this point the athlete may start to feel thirsty; however, by this point the athlete's VO2 MAX decreases by nearly 11 percent, and the blood volume essential for maintaining stroke volume and plasma volume reduces significantly.

Some studies regard hydration status to be the most important factor to be assessed prior to exercise; hydration may be more important than either a fitness or heat acclimatization in determining the athlete's tolerance to exercise in hot climates.

Hydration status is pivotal to peak performance. Water loss from the body can occur through a multitude of ways, but the primary source of fluid loss is from the blood. With dehydration there is inadequate amount of blood left to be pumped throughout the body; this causes an increase in heart rate, because the heart tries to compensate for the low amount of oxygen supplied to the muscles. This leads to a phenomenon known as cardiovascular drift, wherein the heart rate continues to increase, even though the blood output is constant; needless to say that this places an increased stress on the heart muscles.

Dehydration also causes the body to change physiologic pathways: the body tries to preserve blood flow to the muscles by cutting down the blood flow to other regions of the body such as the skin; since the skin is the primary source of thermoregulation and heat dissipation, low blood circulation to the skin causes the heat to be preserved within the body, thus causing the core body temperature to go up; this will ultimately lead to fatigue and improper functioning of the musculoskeletal system.

It is estimated that we lose nearly two-and-a-half cups of water per day simply by evaporation from the skin and by regular breathing. A larger volume of water is dissipated through sweat and urine, and exercise dramatically increases the requirement for water.

Water that is lost through sweat during exercise can amount to 2–6 percent of a person's body weight. [46] Many different factors influence the hydration status of the athlete; these factors include humidity, temperature, activity levels, and the type of clothing the athlete uses during the performance.

Estimating sweat loss:

Each kilogram of weight loss is approximately equal to one liter of fluid deficit. Dividing the total amount of sweat loss by the duration of exercise will provide an estimation of the rate of fluid loss.

One of the easiest ways to monitor sweat loss is by measuring the changes in body mass and then making appropriate adjustments related to fluid intake and urine loss.

For every kilogram of volume consumed during the sport, the athlete may lose about 500 ml of fluid through urine. [30] Each kilogram of weight loss during exercise is equivalent to one liter of fluid deficit.

Instructions for estimating body mass:

The athletes should first weigh themselves in minimal clothing; after the training they should towel dry and take another reading.

How to interpret weight readings (example):

Weight prior to exercise: 70 kg

Weight after exercise: 68 kg

Volume of fluid consumed during exercise = 1 L (one kilogram) minus estimated urine loss (500 ml).

Fluid loss calculations:

Fluid deficit (L): 70 kg - 68 kg = 2 kg

Total sweat loss (L) = 2 Kg + 1 Kg (fluid consumption) - 500 ml (estimated urine loss) = 2.5 kgs

Total exercise duration = 2 hour.

Sweat rate = 2.5/2 = 1.25 L/hr

Below are the estimated rates of sweat loss for athletes from different sporting arenas [30]:

AFL:

Sex	Intensity	Sweat rate (L/h)	Ambient temperature (°C)	Relative humidity (%)
m	-	1.4	12–15	55–88
m	-	1.8	27	52

BASKETBALL:

Sex	Intensity	Sweat rate (L/h)	Ambient temperature (°C)	Relative humidity (%)
m	Competition	1.6	23	41
m	Competition	1.6	19	36
f	Competition	0.9	26	60
f	Competition	1.0	17	58
m	Training	1.4	27	34
m	Training	1.0	20	24
f	Training	0.7	25	43

CYCLING:

Exercise type	Sex	Intensity	Sweat rate (L/h)	Ambient temperature (°C)	Relative humidity (%)
80 min	m	70% VO2max	1.1	20	-
3 hours	m	60% VO2max	1.21	31	22
3 hours (intervals)	m	33-44% VO2max	0.62	33-44	28
2 hours	m	50% VO2max	1.25	30	-
40 km	f	30 km/h	0.75	19-25	-
	m	32 km/h	1.14	19-25	-
1 hour	m	50% VO2max	0.39	25	53
17 min	m	35-45% VO2max	0.29	30	45

ROWING:

Sex	Intensity	Sweat rate (L/h)	Ambient temperature (°C)	Relative humidity (%)
m	Training	2.0	32	-
f	Training	1.4	32	-
m	Training	1.2	10	-
f	Training	0.8	10	-

RUNNING:

Exercise type	Sex	Intensity	Sweat rate (L/h)	Ambient temperature (°C)	Relative humidity (%)
10 km	f	12.8 km/h	1.49	19-24	-
	m	14.6 km/h	1.83	19-24	-
30 km	-	-	1.25	9-17	30-90
2 hours	m	63% VO2max	1.41	22	40-45
42.2 km	-	9.3-15.5 kg/h	1.1	21-26	50-60
	f	9-12 km/h	0.54	6-24	45-85
	m	9-12 km/h	0.81	7	45-85

Exercise type	Sex	Intensity	Sweat rate (L/h)	Ambient temperature (°C)	Relative humidity (%)
	m	8.7–16.1 km/h	0.96	10–12	73
	m	15.9 km/h	1.52	20	37
	-	9.8–15 km/h	0.69-1.27	12–23	-
56 km	-	10.4–14.8 km/h	0.96-1.00	11.3–25.8	-
80 min	m	70% VO2max	1.43	20	-

SOCCER:

Sex	Intensity	Sweat rate (L/h)	Ambient temperature (°C)	Relative humidity (%)
f	Competition	0.8	26	78
m	Competition	1.2	25	41
m	Competition	1.0	10	56
f	Training	0.8	30	35
m	Training	1.0	25	41
m	Training	0.7	9	61
m	-	2.1	33	40
m	-	0.8	13	7
m	-	2.0	13	7
m	-	1.3	19	55

VOLLEYBALL:

Sex	Intensity	Sweat rate (L/h)	Ambient temperature (°C)	Relative humidity (%)
m	Training	0.8	Summer	-
f	Training	0.8	Summer	-

<u>Signs of dehydration:</u>

- Dizziness or lightheadedness

- Nausea or vomiting

- Muscle cramps

- Dry mouth

- Sweating stops

- Heart palpitations

Signs of severe dehydration can include mental confusion, weakness, and loss of consciousness. Seek medical attention immediately if you have any of these symptoms.

Practical strategies for hydration:

1) Consume plenty of fluids the day prior to the event/exercise.

2) Chart your sweat rates during exercise, and adjust your fluid consumption strategy appropriately. It is not necessary to drink enough to prevent loss of body weight, but the amount of dehydration should normally be limited to a loss of less than 2 percent of body weight (e.g., 1.0 kg for 50 kg person, 1.5 kg for a 75 kg person, and 2 kg for a 100 kg person).

3) If you are into endurance sports, then you may want to find a drink that you like the taste of and use it. An electrolyte drink is recommended over plain water because excess consumption of plain water will wash away the electrolytes. Sodium should be included in fluids consumed during exercise lasting longer than one to two hours or during any event that stimulates heavy sodium loss (i.e., more than three to four grams of sodium).

3) Maintain a clean hydration schedule: set up an alarm/reminder that will help you consume the liquids at the adequate time.

4) Monitor your body weight consistently on a daily basis. You may also consider hiring support staff to monitor body weight and UA.

5) Weigh yourself before and after training. If you lose more than 3 percent of your body weight, you need to improve hydration.

6) If you're exercising in a hot environment, it is advisable to find a place that is away from the hot sun and has a cooler temperature; if you're in an outdoor setting, you may choose to practice under the shade.

7) Check for your hydration status regularly prior to the sporting event: pre-exercise hydration status can be assessed from urine frequency and volume, with additional information from urine color, specific gravity, or osmolality. A darker color of urine suggests dehydration.

8) Control body temperature as best you can with proper clothing.

Important tips to consider regarding hydration status:

Do not rely on thirst as the indicator for dehydration; thirst shows up only after 2 percent of water loss (by body weight); by this time it's already too late.

If an athlete has good electrolyte balance prior to the exercise, then water alone is sufficient to maintain good hydration status during short-term exercise that lasts for less than one hour. In case of longer periods of exercise, an electrolyte drink along with carbohydrate and/or carbohydrate with protein supplement will be required to replenish the electrolyte loss.

Always try to maintain adequate hydration prior to the event by consuming more amounts of liquids than required.

The World Health Organization recommends consumption of six to eight large glasses of water per day; however, this is the recommended allowance for regular individuals who do not participate in heavy exercise; therefore, water consumption of more than eight glasses is recommended for athletes.

Guidelines for fluid intake for short-term activities that last less than one hour [47]:

1) Consume adequate fluids throughout the day, and consume approximately two cups of water in the two-hour period prior to exercise.

2) Every fifteen minutes during activity, consume one-half to three-quarter cups of water.

3) Maintain the fluids at a cool temperature (between 59° and 72° F).

4) Use a sports bottle that is convenient to sip from during exercise.

5) Consume approximately two cups of water for every pound lost during exercise (acute shifts in body weight during exercise indicate fluid loss).

6) Avoid dehydrating fluids after exercise; these include coffee, tea, caffeinated sodas, and alcoholic beverages.

For exercise sessions that stretch for more than one hour:

If your exercise extends for more than sixty minutes, you may want to use commercial sports drinks with a carbohydrate content of about 4–8 percent (4–8 g/100 ml) to allow carbohydrate and fluid needs to be met simultaneously.

Take thirty to sixty grams of carbohydrate per hour to delay fatigue and fuel muscle contractions. The intake of carbohydrate that is generally associated with performance benefits is approximately twenty to sixty grams per hour. [31]

Inclusion of sodium (0.5–0.7 g per liter of water) ingested during exercise lasting longer than an hour may improve palatability and therefore encourage athletes to drink more water.

After the exercise:

Health experts recommend [31] drinking 1.2–1.5 liters of fluid for each kilogram of weight lost in training or matches. The most important salt to be consumed is sodium (the main salt lost in sweat) if no food is eaten at this time. Sports drinks that contain electrolytes are helpful, but many foods can also supply the salt that is needed. A little extra salt may be added to meals when sweat losses are high, but salt tablets should be used with caution.

Electrolytes:

What are electrolytes?

Electrolytes are chemicals that form electrically charged particles (ions) in body fluids. These ions carry the electrical energy necessary for many functions, including muscle contractions and transmission of nerve impulses. Many bodily functions depend on electrolytes; optimal performance requires a consistent and adequate supply of these important substances.

Many athletes neglect consistent electrolyte replenishment, because they've never had cramping problems. Even if you've been fortunate enough to have never suffered the painful, debilitating effects of cramping, you still need to provide your body with a consistent and adequate supply of electrolytes. Why? Because the goal of replenishing electrolytes is not to prevent cramping but to maintain specific bodily functions at optimal levels.

Electrolytes are essentially salts; they play a major role in physiology and proper performance.

The most commonly encountered electrolytes in day-to-day life are sodium (Na+), potassium (K+), chloride (cl-), calcium (ca2+) etc.; each of the salts as a negative or positive ion; these ions help in water transport and electrical conductivity in muscular tissues.

Endurolytes by Hammer Nutrition (more information at www.hammernutrition.com):

CALCIUM: Calcium is the most abundant mineral in the human body (about 2.85 lbs/.8 kg in the average person). Normal heart rhythm, healthy nerve transmission, and strong muscle contractions require a constant blood-calcium level. During exercise, calcium-dependent enzymes produce energy from fatty- and amino-acid conversion.

Because fatty acids are such an important fuel during endurance exercise, providing 60–65 percent of your energy needs when exercise goes beyond two hours in length; having adequate calcium available to efficiently convert them into energy is crucial. When blood calcium runs low, the body extracts it from the bones, but this process can't keep up with your exercise depletion rate. Serum calcium deficiency during endurance events may produce high blood pressure, muscle cramps, and weakness.

MAGNESIUM should accompany calcium at a ratio of 1:2. When calcium flows into working muscle cells, the muscle contracts; when calcium leaves and magnesium replaces it, the muscle relaxes. Many enzymatic reactions necessary for fuel conversion to muscular energy occur in the presence of adequate magnesium. Deficiency of magnesium contributes to muscle cramps, tremors, sleep disturbances, and in some cases, convulsive disorders.

POTASSIUM is the chief action (positively charged ion) within all muscle cells. It is necessary for maintaining the optimal concentration and balance of sodium. Potassium deficiency symptoms are nausea, vomiting, muscle weakness, muscle spasms, cramping, and rapid heart rate. Even though 100–200 mg are lost in sweat alone (not counting internal muscle and cell use), if we try to replace those amounts all at once, optimal sodium balance is altered. In addition, too much potassium is hard on the stomach and can cause severe stomach distress.

SODIUM is the chief action (positively charged ion) outside the cell. The average American carries 8,000 mg of excess sodium in extracellular tissues. During endurance events, a minimum of three to four hours is necessary to deplete this mineral, which may result in symptoms of abnormal heartbeat, muscle twitching, and hypoventilation.

However, if sodium is replaced at or near the same rate as depletion, it overrides the hormonal regulating mechanisms that enable the body to conserve electrolytes. Consumption of too much sodium will cause a variety of problems, the least of which is fluid retention. Therefore, we highly recommend a more moderate, body-cooperative replenishment of sodium.

CHLORIDE is the relative anion (negatively charged ion) that accompanies sodium. This electrolyte is absolutely necessary in maintaining the osmotic tension in both blood and extracellular fluids. It's a somewhat complicated process, but to put it in the simplest terms, think of osmotic tension as being the proper balance and consistency of body fluids and electrolytes. An appropriate amount of chloride (as sodium chloride) supports, but does not override, the function of the hormone aldosterone in regulating and conserving proper electrolyte levels.

MANGANESE is included in Endurolytes, as it is necessary in trace amounts for optimal muscle cell enzyme reactions for conversion of fatty acids and protein into energy. Again, fatty acids and protein are a crucial part of the endurance athlete's fuel supply, so, while manganese is not technically an electrolyte, its importance cannot be overstated. Research also shows that manganese deficiency plays a key role in blood-sugar fluctuation, free-radical build-up from intense exercise, and nerve function disorders, especially in older athletes.

PYRIDOXINE HCL (vitamin B-6) is a coenzyme required in sixty enzymatic reactions involving metabolism of carbohydrates, fats, and protein. We include this water-soluble B vitamin in Endurolytes because of its active role in maintaining sodium-potassium balance.

L-TYROSINE is an amino acid added to the Endurolytes formula to protect thyroid and adrenal function. Blood-plasma deficiency during extreme endurance events will lower thyroid and adrenal production, which hinders the proper rate of metabolism. Symptoms of l-tyrosine depletion first appear as depression, later anger, then despondency that degenerates into total despair. If any of these has ever happened to you during a long training session or race, it may be due to low thyroid and adrenal production; it can be easily avoided by the intake of supplemental l-tyrosine via any of the Endurolytes products.

GLYCINE is an amino acid added to Endurolytes Powder to help neutralize the naturally salty/bitter taste of the minerals.

Electrolyte physiology:

Our body has many built-in systems to monitor the hydration and electrolyte balance; these include production of important hormones such as antidiuretic hormone (ADH), parathyroid hormone, and aldosterone to regulate the electrolyte balance.

For example, when the level of blood sodium drops, the kidneys produces hormones that stimulate urine; this in turn reduces the amount of water in the blood and raises the concentration of sodium; on the other hand, if the concentration of sodium is too high, the body produces hormones to stimulate thirst; the subsequent water consumption dilutes the sodium content in blood.

Normal serum electrolyte levels (blood levels)

Sodium, serum: 135–145 mEq/L

Potassium, serum: 3.5–5.0 mEq/L

Chloride, serum: 98–108 mEq/L

Calcium, serum: 8.4–10.2 mEq/dl

Phosphorus, serum: 3.0–4.5 mg/dL

From the above-mentioned levels of electrolytes, it is easy to see that sodium and chloride are the largest electrolytes in blood.

It is estimated that one liter of sweat contains about 1.15g sodium, 0.23g potassium, and 1.48g chloride.

This level is important, because it is not uncommon for a runner or a cyclist to lose one liter of sweat per hour. If you have maintained a good electrolyte balance prior to the exercise, the body will be able to cope with such kinds of electrolyte losses for the first one hour of exercise; however, beyond that, the athlete needs to be supplied with appropriate electrolytes.

Even though sport-drinks companies may want you to believe otherwise, if your exercise period is less than one hour, then you don't need a sports drink; all you need is water. Sipping water throughout the workout will be adequate to get through the workout.

Important note: athletes who participate in events conducted in dry environments tend to experience lower levels of sweating; this is because the low humidity (dry atmosphere) causes sweat to evaporate quickly, which leads to dehydration; if the athlete does not understand this concept, he or she may not consume adequate fluids simply because of not sweating; this may lead to significant dehydration.

Natural sources of electrolytes:

Electrolyte content of some foods: mg of electrolytes contained per 100 g / 3.5 oz of food			
100g	mg. Na	Cl	K
Milk	55	100	139
Wheat flour (whole)	2	38	290
Rice (polished, raw)	6	27	110
Potatoes	3	79	410
Carrots	50	69	311
Apricots	0.6	—	440
Dates (dried)	1	290	790
Oranges	1	3	170
Bread (whole meal)	540	860	220
Bananas	1	93	467

Snacks that replenish electrolyte balance:

1) A combination of nuts (salted peanuts) and raisins. Nuts have high levels of protein, sodium, and fats, whereas raisins contain carbohydrates and potassium; these two ingredients can serve as a good electrolyte snack.

2) Watermelon, honeydew, cantaloupe, and other such fruits and vegetables are excellent sources of water, sugar, and electrolytes.

Ingredients for homemade sports drinks (1 liter):

1) Half a teaspoon of table salt in two liters of water makes a good electrolyte drink.

2) Pure fruit juice concentrate (200–240 ml or 8 oz) without any added sugars + water or green tea (to 1 liter) + salt (1/3–1/2 teaspoon)

3) Chicken and vegetable broth also serve as good electrolyte replacements.

Rules for electrolyte consumption:

1) Electrolyte supplements are not required for the first hour.

2) An athlete may lose around 1 g of sodium per hour via sweat; however, it is important to remember that all of this electrolyte need not be replaced, attempting to do so will result in overload and intolerance, leading to symptoms such as gastrointestinal distress, nausea, vomiting, or diarrhea.

3) If the period of exercise extends for more than one hour, it would be beneficial for the athlete to consume at least .5 to 1 L of water per hour with 500 mg of sodium/liter.

4) It's important to remember that 1 teaspoon of table salt contains nearly 2,500 mg of sodium.

5) The athlete may also choose to consume a sports drink that contains electrolytes such as potassium, magnesium, and calcium.

Management of dehydration in sports:

The following table provides information to help determine the hydration status and electrolyte adjustments required for endurance athletes. The table consists of various states such as hydration low, hydration OK, hydration high, and electrolytes low, OK, and high.

This table serves as a quick reference chart for athletes and sports trainers.

This table first appeared in the May 2007 issue of *UltraRunning Magazine* and was created by Karl King; since then it's been used as a quick reference table to assess the electrolyte and hydration balance.

	Hydration LOW	Hydration OK	Hydration HIGH
Electrolytes HIGH	Hypernatremia with dehydration Likelihood: moderate Weight is down a few pounds or more. Thirst is high, and salty foods taste bad. Mouth and skin are dry. Food acceptance is poor. Absence of urination. **Causes:** no access to water or voluntary restriction of water intake; body electrolytes concentrated by loss of water. **What to do:** get access to water and drink. Restrict electrolytes until weight is near normal.	Hypernatremia Likelihood: rare, transitory if water available Weight is normal. Thirst is high, and salty foods taste bad. Mouth is not very dry. **Causes:** no access to water, or voluntary restriction of water intake; body electrolytes concentrated by loss of water. **What to do:** drink to satisfy thirst, so that excess electrolytes are removed by sweating and urination. Restrict salt intake until excess is urinated and sweated out.	Hypernatremia with over-hydration Likelihood: very rare Weight is up a few pounds or more Thirst is high, and salty foods taste bad. Possible mental confusion; hands may be puffy; shortness of breath; rapid heart rate. Food acceptance is poor. **Causes:** overconsumption of salt, probably from a combination of sources **What to do:** stop electrolyte intake; drink only to wet mouth until weight is normal.

	Hydration LOW	Hydration OK	Hydration HIGH
Electrolytes OK	Dehydration	Proper hydration and electrolyte balance	Overhydrated
	Likelihood: common	Likelihood: common	Likelihood: moderate
	Weight is down a few pounds or more.	Weight is stable or slightly down.	Weight is up a few pounds or more.
	Thirst is high, and salty foods taste normal. Mouth is dry; food acceptance is poor.	Stomach is fine; food acceptance is normal. Mouth is moist (can spit), and skin is normal. Cramps: none. Urination is normal.	Wrists and hands are probably puffy.
	Skin is dry and may tent if pinched.		Stomach is queasy.
	May have dizziness on standing up		Thirst is low, and salty foods taste normal.
	May have cramping Mental performance may be affected.		Mouth is moist; can spit.
	Causes: insufficient fluid intake	**Causes**: proper water and electrolyte intake	**Causes**: fluid intake in excess of needs
	What to do: drink sports drink with electrolytes, or water.	**What to do**: continue with hydration and electrolyte practice unless conditions change.	**What to do**: drink only to wet mouth until weight is near normal.

	Hydration LOW	Hydration OK	Hydration HIGH
Electrolytes LOW	Hyponatremia with dehydration	Hyponatremia	Hyponatremia with overhydration; dangerous!
	Likelihood: rare	Likelihood: mild form is common.	Likelihood: moderate
	Weight is down a few pounds or more.	Weight is normal.	Weight is up a few pounds or more.
	Thirst is high, and salty foods taste good.	Stomach is queasy, with poor food acceptance.	Wrists and hands are puffy.
	Mouth is dry; can't spit.	Wrists may be puffy.	Nausea, stomach sloshing, possible vomiting. Thirst is low, and salty foods taste very good.
	May have cramping.	Salty foods taste good.	Athlete may show mental confusion, odd behavior.
	Skin is dry and may tent if pinched.	Thirst is normal.	Mouth is moist—can spit.
	May have dizziness on standing up	Mouth is moist—can spit.	Urination may be voluminous and crystal-clear.
	Causes: insufficient drinking, no electrolyte intake	May have cramping	**Causes:** overhydration, insufficient sodium intake
	What to do: take electrolytes and drink sports drink or water.	**Causes:** insufficient electrolyte intake	**What to do:** drink only to wet mouth until weight is normal, then correct any sodium deficit.
		What to do: increase electrolyte intake until stomach feels OK.	

Carbohydrates in sport:

Why are carbohydrates important for athletes?

Your muscle cells are most sensitive to insulin during the first hour after exercise. Assuming that enough carbohydrates are available, elevated levels of insulin in the blood after exercise speed up the transport of glucose into your muscle cells.

Clinical studies have shown that athletes who waited more than one hour to consume carbohydrates restored about 50 percent less muscle glycogen than did athletes who consumed carbohydrates during the period of maximum insulin sensitivity.

You need to replenish your liver and muscle glycogen stores to the optimal amount as soon as possible to speed the recovery process.

The principal glucose transporter protein that mediates this uptake is glucose transporter type 4 (GLUT4), which plays a key role in regulating whole-body glucose homeostasis.

We actually know that there is a two-phase process of glycogen replenishment. The first phase begins immediately after the exercise; the second phase is a slower but longer-lasting process in which carbohydrate-hungry muscles become more sensitive to insulin (the anabolic hormone that drives the glucose into cells).

What do we need carbohydrates for?

Here's a brief walkthrough of how carbohydrates help us perform at optimal levels:

Our brain/nerve cells use nearly 7 g of carbohydrates per hour to function at an optimal rate, so we would need about 168 g of carbohydrates per day to use our brain and nervous system; however, 50 percent of this carbohydrate load is generated from gluconeogenesis; therefore, we need to consume about 84 g of carbohydrate per day.

Total amount of carbohydrate used for other functions amounts to 125–150 g per day.

Therefore we need to consume a total of 210 to 235 g of carbohydrates per day to function normally (for sedentary life).

Extra physical activities consume extra carbohydrates:

- 30 minutes of easy walking = about 25 g

- 45 minutes of moderate running = about 75 g

- 60 minutes of hard running = 125 g

- 120 minutes of interval running = 200 g

We always carry a reserve of carbohydrates in the form of glycogen stored in the liver, muscle tissue, and circulating blood glucose.

An average 70 kg (154.3 lbs) male has 1500–1600 kcal of carbohydrate reserve.

- Muscle stores: 1200 kcal = 30 g

- Liver stores: 320 kcal = 80 g

- Blood glucose: 20 kcal = 5 g

Suggested carbohydrate (CHO) intake ranges of 5 to 7 g/kg/day for general training needs and 7 to 10 g/kg/day for the increased needs of endurance athletes are suggested. [51]

For an average athlete weighing 70 kgs, this would amount to 350–490 g/day (1400–1960 kcal) of carbohydrate for general training needs and 490 to 700 g/day (1960–2800 kcal) of carbohydrates for the increased needs of endurance athletes.

This implies that nearly 55–60 percent of the daily calories should be derived from carbohydrates for optimal performance.

Benefits of carbohydrate feeding:

1) *Increased endurance and performance*: Numerous studies conducted on carbohydrate feeding during exercise have provided convincing evidence that any athlete exercising for forty-five minutes or longer can benefit from carbohydrate feeding.

Studies have demonstrated that a drop in blood glucose can be prevented by carbohydrate feeding during exercise at 70 percent of V.O2max. [49].

It's been found that participants who are able to maintain glucose concentrations above 3 mmol/L through carbohydrate feeding can exercise for up to four hours at the same intensity, whereas the same effect is not noticed in the subjects who consumed only water or placebo. [49]

2) *Glycogen-sparing effect*: As discussed earlier in the book, carbohydrate feeding produces a glycogen-sparing function in the liver and muscle tissue.

3) *Glycogen synthesis*: Carbohydrate feeding also promotes glycogen synthesis during exercise; research studies have demonstrated that muscle glycogen concentrations are higher after intermittent exercise when carbohydrate was ingested instead of water. [50]

4) *Improved sensory function*: It's been found that carbohydrates may affect the central nervous system in the form of mood change, better perception, and judgment. The opposite effect may be observed in a hypoglycemic person.

5) Studies by Costill et al. showed that runners consuming 40 percent of energy from CHO could not replenish muscle glycogen on a daily basis, whereas runners on a 70 percent CHO diet could.

How to improve athletic performance by increasing muscle glycogen stores:

We discussed earlier that glycogen stored in muscles can be used for generating energy required for extreme athletic performance. The amount of glycogen stored in muscles prior to an athletic event can be increased by modifying the diet and exercise routines through a plan known as *super-compensation.*

There are two typical approaches to super-compensation
1. Depletion/repletion:
This process involves maximum depletion of glycogen reserves through an extremely long duration of exercise about seven to ten days prior to the major competition, followed by a few days of very low-CHO diet. This is supplement by a second bout of long exercise four days prior to competition and then three days of a high-CHO diet.

Benefits:

- Muscle glycogen stores can be greatly increased, often by as much as 50 percent over the usual "full" condition (e.g., from 300 → over 400 grams).

- If it costs 100 kcal to run a mile, and 60 percent of energy comes from muscle glycogen = 60 kcal of glycogen mile = 15 g glycogen needed/mile. If you start with 300 g, you can run twenty miles before running out.

- If you increase to 400 g, you can extend run to 26.5 miles.

2. Modified moderate approach:

This is a more popular approach; the athlete begins to taper the training one week prior to the competition date and simultaneously increases the percentage of carbohydrates in the diet (e.g., from 50–60 percent up to 70–75 percent).

It's important to note that the increases in muscle glycogen are not as dramatic as with the depletion/repletion method; an increase of up to 20 percent of stored muscle glycogen can be expected with this method.

Benefits of carbohydrate loading:

- A higher amount of reserve glycogen increases time to exhaustion.

- Higher reserves of glycogen also reduce the time to complete a task.

- It may also improve performance in team sports that require intermittent exercise and skill executions.

Disadvantages of carbohydrate loading:

This benefit can be experienced only over one day of exercise; it may not be beneficial for athletes involved in consecutive days of competition.

Carbohydrates are mostly stored along with water; every gram of carbohydrate usually retains about 3 g of water; therefore, when glycogen storage is increased by 200 g, the expected weight gain would be around 800 g (200 g glycogen + 600 g water).

What should you consume during the event?

1) Select a glucose polymer. (Gatorade is good.)

2) Avoid simple sugars such as galactose and fructose that are available in the form of fruit juices and plain sugar drinks/sugar bars; these must first be converted to glucose by the liver to be used as a substrate.

3) As mentioned earlier, choose drinks ranging from 4–8% CHO. Drinks with too much CHO (Coke has 11.25% CHO) will not be absorbed as efficiently and could cause stomach upset.

Recommended rate of carbohydrate feeding after exercise:

From 1 to 1.85 g per kg of body weight per hour after exercise, and at fifteen- to sixty-minute intervals thereafter, for up to five hours.

Protein:

Proteins are considered the building blocks of our body. Our muscles, tendons, hair, skin, and other tissues are made up of proteins; they not only help in structural support, but they also help in enzyme production and nutrient transfer. Proteins are made up of various types of amino acids; it's estimated that the body contains nearly ten thousand different types of proteins.

It is important to note that protein cannot be easily stored by our body; therefore, it is vital to consume protein at regular intervals.

For protein to serve as a building block, it needs to contain all the essential amino acids; most of these amino acids can be found in animal foods such as eggs, fish, meat, etc.

Vegetable sources do not provide all the essential amino acids required for muscle building and recovery; for this reason it is very important for vegetarian athletes to learn how to combine foods to get all the essential amino acids.

Why do athletes need more proteins?

Athletes are continuously stretching their endurance limits; needless to say, this leads to muscle wear and tear; the body faces a constant demand to repair itself, and this process requires proteins.

Proteins also help carbohydrate loading and storing, so carbohydrates can be used as ready fuel during the competition. It's important to note that protein may not be the ideal source of fuel for exercise; however, it aids in muscle building and recovery.

Recommended daily protein intake:

- The average adult needs 0.8 grams per kilogram (2.2 lbs) of body weight per day.

- Strength-training athletes need about 1.4 to 1.8 grams per kilogram (2.2 lbs) of body weight per day.

- Research supports a range in protein needs from 1.2 to 1.4 grams of protein per kilogram body weight for endurance athletes such as marathoners. [42, 43]

It's easy to get the daily protein requirements, because protein is found in most foods:

- Meat, poultry, and fish: 7 grams per ounce

- Beans, dried peas, and lentils: 7 grams per 1/2 cup cooked

- One large egg: 7 grams

- Milk: 8 grams per cup

- Bread: 4 grams per slice

- Cereal: 4 grams per 1/2 cup

- Vegetables: 2 grams per 1/2 cup

In this section, let's have a quick look at the guidelines for intake of protein supplements:

1) Consume 15 to 25 g of protein within the first hour after exercise to begin repair.

2) You can enhance the insulin response in your body by adding proteins and carbohydrates.

3) It is important to remember that protein may not be the ideal snack prior to exercise, because it stimulates the production of a substance known as cholecystokinin (CCK), which slows the rate of gastric emptying and fluid absorption.

Recommended supplements:

- R4 system by Ed Burke: 4:1 carbs to protein ration

- Power Bar Recovery: 6.25:1 carbs to protein

- Gatorade Recovery: .825:1 carbs to protein

- Hammer Nutrition Recovery: 3:1 carbs to protein

- Herbal 24 Life Formula One: 1.44 carbs to protein

- Herbal 24 Life Rebuild Endurance: 1.44 carbs to protein

- Herbal 24 Life Rebuild Strength: .58 carbs to protein

Whey protein releases its amino acids much sooner than other forms of protein; therefore, a dose of whey protein (shake) consumed quickly after exercise can enhance the rate of protein synthesis and recovery.

Additional elements to monitor:

- **Anabolic** processes tend toward "building up" organs and tissues. These processes produce growth and differentiation of cells and increase in body size, a process that involves synthesis of complex molecules. Examples of anabolic processes include the growth and mineralization of bone and increases in muscle mass. The hormone involved in the anabolic process is testosterone.

- **Catabolism** (Greek *kata* = downward + *ballein* = to throw) is the set of metabolic pathways that breaks down molecules into smaller units and releases energy. In catabolism, large molecules such as polysaccharides, lipids, nucleic acids, and proteins are broken down into smaller units such as monosaccharides, fatty acids, nucleotides, and amino acids, respectively. The hormone involved in the catabolic process is cortisol. The effects of cortisol have been discussed in details in the chapter on stress (p. 26).

RecoveryDoc Recommendation for protein intake via supplements

- Power Sports

  Morning: Consume Whey Protein Shake with milk; total calories based on athlete's weight and sport.

  Workout: Immediately after workout consume Whey Protein Shake; at thirty minutes consume 1:1 or greater recovery drink.

  At bedtime consume Casein Protein Shake with water, not milk.

- Endurance:

  Morning: Consume Whey Protein Shake based on the season and the weight of athlete.

  Workout: Immediately after workout consume 5:1 or greater recovery drink; at bedtime consume Casein Protein Shake.

The pre-workout meal:

The pre-workout meal has a major impact on the intensity of your workout. Research studies [32] have revealed that the exercise intensity, pace, and work output decrease as glycogen levels diminish; therefore, it is important to ensure that your body has enough energy and fuel to meet the demands of the exercise. The right nutrition consumed at the right time can help you gain muscle mass, recover faster, increase your energy levels, and even improve your performance!

An intense workout contributes only a minor proportion to your overall athletic endurance; however, your nutrition can have a make-or-break effect on your overall progress. A good diet supplied at the right time fuels the molecular process responsible for growth and recovery.

The International Society of Sports Nutrition (ISSN) recommends eating a meal about two to four hours before you train. The ideal meal would consist of protein and low-glycemic index (GI) carbohydrates as well as water for hydration. Kerksick et al. (2008) noted that "regular ingestion of various protein sources in conjunction with carbohydrate stimulates greater increases in strength and favorably impacts body composition when compared to carbohydrate alone." The selected foods should be low in fat, be familiar to the player's digestive system, and should be consumed close enough to a workout in order to promote faster gastric emptying and reduced chances of gastric distress.

During the workout:

Hydration is very important during workout. Your pre-workout meal supplies you with the energy needed to get through your workout; your main goal during the workout will be to replace the fluid lost and to provide carbohydrates for maintenance of blood sugar (glucose) levels. The recommended rate of fluid consumption is drinking about 8 oz every fifteen minutes.

If your exercise regimen is longer than sixty minutes, then 30–60 g of carbohydrate per hour should be consumed in order to maintain blood glucose and muscle glycogen stores. [35] According to some experts, [33] a 6–8 percent carbohydrate solution is recommended to replenish glycogen stores and electrolytes.

Post-workout meal:

After you get through the training process, it is important to focus on the recovery and try to replenish all your energy stores. The first thirty minutes after a workout is described as the golden anabolic window, since maximum results can be achieved by the athlete if the right foods are consumed during this period.

Inadequate recovery can limit an athlete's success; if the athlete waits for too long to consume a post-workout meal, it will have profound negative effects on athletic function.

The ideal post-workout meal should consist of high-GI carbohydrates and highly absorbable protein (such as whey protein in powder form) in a 3:1 (carbs to protein) ratio. [34] These high-GI carbs will initiate a rapid rise in blood sugar, which will in turn stimulate an insulin release and lead to subsequent absorption of fluids and nutrients into muscle and body cells.

This post-workout snack must be followed up with a larger meal that is to be eaten about two hours later. This well-balanced meal should consist of a generous serving of lean protein, complex carbohydrate, a moderate amount of fat, and as many vegetables as you wish.

Testosterone to cortisol ratio:

Cortisol is one of the major hormones released by the adrenal gland in response to strenuous physical exercise. It's been found that if an athlete fails to follow appropriate measures for recovery after strenuous exercise, he or she will experience high levels of cortisol, which can subsequently lead to fatigue, loss of lean muscle, and reduced performance.

Testosterone is responsible for enhanced physical performance and anabolic muscle growth. Low levels of testosterone have been linked to reduced lean body muscle and a higher risk of osteoporosis.

The ratio:

The testosterone to cortisol ratio (fTC) is the ratio of blood levels of unbound or free testosterone and cortisol in their molar concentrations.

A low testosterone cortisol ratio serves as an indicator for overtraining and signifies muscle breakdown, poor physical performance, and an increased catabolic state in athletes.

Researchers [36] suggest that a 30 percent or more decrease in fTC may suggest an inappropriate level of anabolic to catabolic hormonal balance.

The metabolic effects of testosterone and cortisol are depicted in the diagram below: [37]

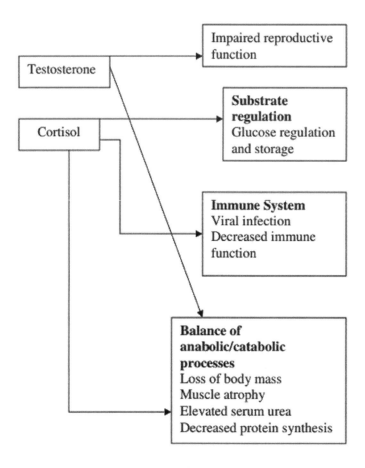

Significance: a regular analysis of testosterone cortisol ratio can serve as a real-time indicator for recovery rates in athletes.

Eating Habits: Create a clean and healthy diet:

1. Avoid artificial sweeteners: Many sugar substitutes:

The four major groups of FDA-approved artificial sweeteners on the market are

- Aspartame (includes Equal, Nutrasweet brands),

- Sucralose (includes Splenda brand),

- Saccharin (includes Sweet'N Low brand), and

- Acesulfame potassium (includes Sunett, Sweet One brands).

Artificial sweeteners are linked to several health issues; some researchers are of the opinion that artificial sweeteners may stimulate the taste-bud receptors and thereby cause an increase in insulin; for this reason, it is best to substitute artificial sweeteners with natural sweeteners such as xylitol.

2. Avoid high-fructose corn syrup: Corn-based syrup is used in many products. Even though corn is healthy in its natural form, high-fructose corn syrup is notorious for raising the blood sugar much faster than other forms of sweeteners or sugars; therefore, it is best to avoid foods with high-fructose corn syrup. Make sure you read the labels of foods to see if this ingredient is included.

3. Avoid artificial food colors: It's estimated that Americans are now eating five times as much food dyes as they did in 1955. Health experts from FDA now suspect certain food dyes (Red 40 & Yellow 5) are linked to hyperactivity in children.

Here are some strategies to avoid artificial food dyes:

Eat more organic food: Many foods carry the label "made with organic ingredients"; however, they may still contain synthetic dyes; for this reason it is important to ignore manufacturer claims and look for organic foods with the green and white USDA label that certifies organic foods.

Opt for natural colors: Beet, carotenes, annatto, or capsanthin (capsicum extract) are natural colors—look if these ingredients are present on the labels of colored foods.

Look for colors with a number code: Synthetic colors carry a number code next to them (Red 40, Green 3, Blue 1 and 2). Avoid these.

"Artificial colors" label does not necessarily mean synthetic: Artificial color represents both natural and synthetic colors—it signifies that the colors were not naturally present in these ingredients, and hence another substitute was used (it could be natural or synthetic). If a synthetic element was used, it will be mentioned in the label with a color and number code.

4. Avoid soda: It is estimated that the average American consumes about fifty-three gallons of soda per year—these sodas contain several chemicals and sweeteners that can raise blood-sugar levels instantly and also cause damage to your teeth.

5. Make sure all your foods are well cooked: Boiling food at high temperatures kills bacteria and fungi.

6. Choose organic foods: Many food producers nowadays take advantage of freely available hormones to produce vegetables that are high on quantity but low on nutrients. Organic foods are grown naturally without any artificial hormones; for this reason they are more nutritious.

7. Wash and clean your foods before you eat: Many pesticides and fertilizers are used by farmers to improve the harvest; these chemical substances will stick to the plants to help them grow faster without insect infestation; these foods don't go through a washing process after they are harvested. For this reason it is important to soak fresh vegetables in water and give them a thorough wash before using them.

8. Wash first, cut later: Cutting vegetable exposes their fleshy, nutrient-filled inner regions; washing foods after cutting them will cause the nutrients to be washed away from the exposed regions; for this reason it is important to wash the vegetables before cutting them and not vice versa.

9. Become excellent at reading food labels: Below is a detailed explanation on how to read food labels and nutrition components; it's worth spending some time to understand all the components of food labels, because this knowledge will serve you lifelong.

The Nutrition Facts label—an overview:

The following section contains official guidelines from the FDA on reading food and nutrition labels:

(To read more go to http://www.fda.gov/food/ResourcesForYou/Consumers/NFLPM/ucm274593.htm.)

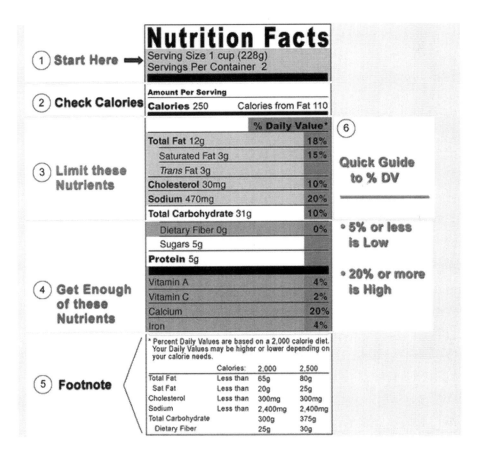

The information in the main or top section (see numbers 1–4 and number 6 on the sample nutrition label above) can vary with each food product; it contains product-specific information (serving size, calories, and nutrient information). The bottom part (see number 5 on the sample label above) contains a footnote with daily values (DVs) for 2,000- and 2,500-calorie diets. This footnote provides recommended dietary information for important nutrients, including fats, sodium, and fiber.

The footnote is found only on larger packages and does not change from product to product.

In the following Nutrition Facts label, we have colored certain sections to help you focus on those areas that will be explained in detail. You will not see these colors on the food labels on products you purchase.

① The serving size:

Serving Size 1 cup (228g)
Servings Per Container 2

The first place to start when you look at the Nutrition Facts label is the serving size and the number of servings in the package. Serving sizes are standardized to make it easier to compare similar foods; they are provided in familiar units, such as cups or pieces, followed by the metric amount (e.g., the number of grams).

The size of the serving on the food package influences the number of calories and all the nutrient amounts listed on the top part of the label. *Pay attention to the serving size*, especially how many servings there are in the food package. Then ask yourself, *"How many servings am I consuming?"* (e.g., 1/2 serving, 1 serving, or more) In the sample label, one serving of macaroni and cheese equals one cup. If you ate the whole package, you would eat *two* cups. That doubles the calories and other nutrient numbers, including the percentage of daily values as shown in the sample label.

Example				
	Single Serving	**%DV**	**Double Serving**	**%DV**
Serving Size	1 cup (228g)		2 cups (456g)	
Calories	250		500	
Calories from Fat	110		220	
Total Fat	12g	18%	24g	36%
Trans Fat	1.5g		3g	
Saturated Fat	3g	15%	6g	30%
Cholesterol	30mg	10%	60mg	20%
Sodium	470mg	20%	940mg	40%
Total Carbohydrate	31g	10%	62g	20%
Dietary Fiber	0g	0%	0g	0%
Sugars	5g		10g	
Protein	5g		10g	
Vitamin A		4%		8%
Vitamin C		2%		4%
Calcium		20%		40%
Iron		4%		8%

② Calories (and calories from fat):

Calories provide a measure of how much energy you get from a serving of this food. Many Americans consume more calories than they need without meeting recommended intakes for a number of nutrients. The calorie section of the label can help you manage your weight (i.e., gain, lose, or maintain). *The number of servings* you eat *determines the number of calories you actually consume* (your portion amount).

Amount Per Serving	
Calories 250	Calories from Fat 110

In the above example, there are 250 calories in one serving of this macaroni and cheese. How many calories from fat are there in *one* serving? Answer: 110 calories, which means almost half the calories in a single serving come from fat. What if you ate the whole package's contents? Then you would consume two servings, or 500 calories, and 220 would come from fat.

General guide to calories:

- 40 calories is low

- 100 calories is moderate

- 400 calories or more is high

The above guide to calories provides a general reference for calories when you look at a Nutrition Facts label. This guide is based on a 2,000-calorie diet.

Eating too many calories per day is linked to *overweight* and *obesity*.

③④ The nutrients: How much?

Look at the top of the nutrient section in the sample label. It shows you some key nutrients that impact your health and separates them into two main groups.

Limit These Nutrients:

(#3 on sample label):

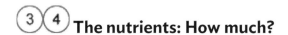

Total Fat 12g	18%
Saturated Fat 3g	15%
Trans Fat 3g	
Cholesterol 30mg	10%
Sodium 470mg	20%

The nutrients listed first are the ones Americans generally eat in adequate amounts, or even too much. They are identified in yellow as *Limit These Nutrients*. Eating too much fat, saturated fat, *trans* fat, cholesterol, or sodium may increase your risk of certain chronic diseases, such as heart disease, some cancers, or high blood pressure.

Important: Health experts recommend that you keep your intake of saturated fat, *trans* fat, and cholesterol as low as possible as part of a nutritionally balanced diet.

Get enough of these:

(#4 on sample label):

Dietary Fiber 0g	0%
Vitamin A	4%
Vitamin C	2%
Calcium	20%
Iron	4%

Most Americans don't get enough dietary fiber, vitamin A, vitamin C, calcium, and iron in their diets. They are identified in blue as *Get Enough of These Nutrients*. Eating enough of these nutrients can improve your health and help reduce the risk of some diseases and conditions.

For example, getting enough calcium may reduce the risk of osteoporosis, a condition that results in brittle bones as one ages (see calcium section below). Eating a diet high in dietary fiber promotes healthy bowel function. Additionally, a diet rich in fruits, vegetables, and grain products that contain dietary fiber (particularly soluble fiber) and low in saturated fat and cholesterol may reduce the risk of heart disease.

Remember: You can use the Nutrition Facts label not only to help *limit* those nutrients you want to cut back on but also to *increase* those nutrients you need to consume in greater amounts.

(5) **Understanding the footnote on the bottom of the Nutrition Facts label:**

Note the asterisk used after the heading *% Daily Value* on the Nutrition Facts label. It refers to the Footnote in the lower part of the nutrition label, which tells you "Percent daily values are based on a 2,000 calorie diet." This statement must be on all food labels.

But the remaining information in the full footnote may not be on the package if the size of the label is too small. When the full footnote does appear, it will always be the same. It doesn't change from product to product, because it shows general recommended dietary advice for all Americans—it is not about a specific food product.

Look at the amounts circled in red in the footnote—these are the DVs for each nutrient listed and are based on public-health experts' advice. DVs are recommended levels of intakes. DVs in the footnote are based on a 2,000- or 2,500-calorie diet. Note how the DVs for some nutrients change, while others (for cholesterol and sodium) remain the same for both calorie amounts.

How the Daily Values relate to the %DVs:

Look at the example below for another way to see how the DVs relate to the percent of DVs and dietary guidance. For each nutrient listed, there is a column labeled *DV*, *%DV*, and *goal* or dietary advice. If you follow this dietary advice, you will stay within public health experts' recommended upper or lower limits for the nutrients listed, based on a 2,000-calorie daily diet.

Examples of DVs versus %DVs:
Based on a 2,000 Calorie Diet:

Nutrient	DV	%DV	Goal
Total Fat	65g	= 100%DV	Less than
Sat Fat	20g	= 100%DV	Less than
Cholesterol	300mg	= 100%DV	Less than
Sodium	2400mg	= 100%DV	Less than
Total Carbohydrate	300g	= 100%DV	At least
Dietary Fiber	25g	= 100%DV	At least

Upper limit—eating "Less than":

The nutrients that have "upper daily limits" are listed first on the foot-note of larger labels and on the example above. Upper limits means it is recommended that you stay below—eat "less than"—the DV nutrient amounts listed per day. For example, the DV for saturated fat (in the yellow section) is 20 g. This amount is 100 percent of the DV for this nutrient. What is the goal or dietary advice? To eat less than 20 g or 100 percent of the DV for the day.

Lower limit—eating "At least":

Now look at the section in blue where dietary fiber is listed. The DV for dietary fiber is 25 g, which is 100 percent of the DV. This means it is recommended that you eat *at least* this amount of dietary fiber per day.

The DV for total carbohydrate (section in white) is 300 g or 100 percent of DV. This amount is recommended for a balanced daily diet that is based on 2,000 calories, but can vary, depending on your daily intake of fat and protein.

Now let's look at the column headed *%DV*s.

⑥ The percent daily value (%DV):

The percent daily values (%DVs) are based on the daily value recommendations for key nutrients but only for a 2,000-calorie daily diet—not 2,500 calories. You, like most people, may not know how many calories you consume in a day. But you can still use the %DV as a frame of reference whether you consume more or less than 2,000 calories.

The %DV helps you determine if a serving of food is high or low in a nutrient. Note: a few nutrients, like *trans* fat, do not have a %DV—they will be discussed later.

Do you need to know how to calculate percentages to use the %DV? No; the label (the %DV) does the math for you. It helps you interpret the numbers (grams and milligrams) by putting them all on the same scale for the day (0–100%DV). The %DV column doesn't add up vertically to 100 percent. Instead each nutrient is based on 100 percent of the daily requirements for that nutrient (for a 2,000-calorie diet). This way you can tell high from low and know which nutrients contribute a lot, or a little, to your *daily* recommended allowance (upper or lower).

Quick Guide to %DV:

	% Daily Value*
Total Fat 12g	18%
Saturated Fat 3g	15%
Trans Fat 3g	
Cholesterol 30mg	10%
Sodium 470mg	20%
Total Carbohydrate 31g	10%
Dietary Fiber 0g	0%
Sugars 5g	
Protein 5g	
Vitamin A	4%
Vitamin C	2%
Calcium	20%
Iron	4%

Up to 5%DV is low and 20%DV or more is high for all nutrients, those you want to limit (e.g., fat, saturated fat, cholesterol, and sodium), and for those that you want to consume in greater amounts (fiber, calcium, etc.).

Example: Look at the amount of total fat in one serving listed on the sample nutrition label. Is 18%DV contributing a lot or a little to your fat limit of 100%DV? Check the *Quick Guide to %DV*. 18%DV, which is below 20%DV, is not yet high, but what if you ate the whole package (two servings)? You would double that amount, eating 36 percent of your daily allowance for total fat. Coming from just one food, that amount leaves you with 64 percent of your fat allowance

(100% - 36% = 64%) for *all* of the other foods you eat that day, snacks and drinks included.

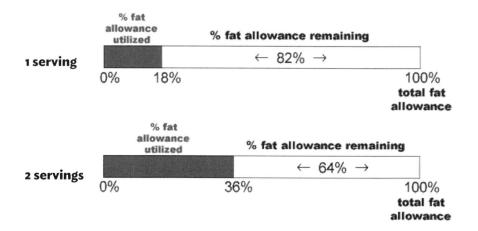

Using the %DV for the following:

Comparisons: The %DV also makes it easy for you to make comparisons. You can compare one product or brand to a similar product. Just make sure the serving sizes are similar, especially the weight (e.g., gram, milligram, ounces) of each product. It's easy to see which foods are higher or lower in nutrients, because the serving sizes are generally consistent for similar types of foods (see the comparison example at the end), except in a few cases like cereals.

Nutrient Content Claims: Use the %DV to help you quickly distinguish one claim from another, such as "reduced fat" vs. "light" or "nonfat." Just compare the %DVs for total fat in each food product to see which one is higher or lower in that nutrient—*there is no need to memorize definitions.* This works when comparing all nutrient content claims (e.g., *less, light, low, free, more,* or *high*).

Dietary trade-offs: You can *use the %DV to help you make dietary trade-offs* with other foods throughout the day. You don't have to give up a favorite food to eat a healthy diet. When a food you like is high in fat, balance it with foods that are low in fat at other times of the day. Also, pay attention to how much you eat, so that the *total* amount of fat for the day stays below 100%DV.

Nutrients with a %DV but no weight listed—spotlight on calcium:

```
Nutrition Facts
Serving Size 1 cup (236ml)
Servings Per Container 1

Amount Per Serving
Calories 80       Calories from Fat 0
                              % Daily Value*
Total Fat  0g                        0%
  Saturated Fat 0g                   0%
  Trans Fat 0g
Cholesterol  Less than 5mg           0%
Sodium  120mg                        5%
Total Carbohydrate 11g               4%
  Dietary Fiber 0g                   0%
  Sugars 11g
Protein  9g                         17%

Vitamin A 10%      •     Vitamin C 4%
Calcium 30% • Iron 0% • Vitamin D 25%
*Percent Daily Values are based on a 2,000
calorie diet. Your daily values may be higher
or lower depending on your calorie needs.
```

Calcium: Look at the %DV for calcium on food packages, so you know how much one serving contributes to the *total amount you need* per day. Remember, a food with 20%DV or more contributes a lot of calcium to your daily total, while one with 5%DV or less contributes a little.

Experts advise adult consumers to consume adequate amounts of calcium; that is, 1,000 mg or 100%DV in a daily 2,000-calorie diet. This advice is often given in milligrams (mg), but the Nutrition Facts label *only* lists a %DV for calcium.

For certain populations, they advise that adolescents, especially girls, consume 1,300 mg (130%DV) and post-menopausal women consume 1,200 mg (120%DV) of calcium daily. The DV for calcium on food labels is 1,000 mg.

Don't be fooled—always check the label for calcium, because you can't make assumptions about the amount of calcium in specific food categories. For example, the amount of calcium in milk, whether skim or whole, is generally the same per serving, whereas the amount of calcium in the same size yogurt container (8 oz) can vary from 20–45%DV.

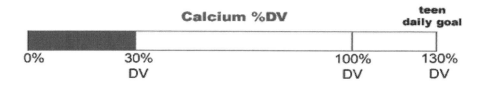

Equivalencies:

30%DV = 300 mg calcium = one cup of milk

100%DV = 1,000 mg calcium

130%DV = 1,300 mg calcium

Nutrients without a %DV: Trans fats, protein, and sugars:

Note that *trans* fat, sugars, and protein do not list a %DV on the Nutrition Facts label.

Plain Yogurt

Fruit Yogurt

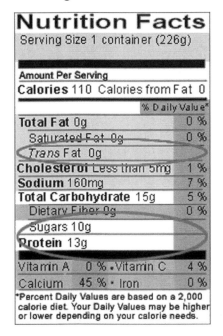

Trans fat: Experts could not provide a reference value for *trans* fat nor any other information that FDA believes is sufficient to establish a Daily Value or %DV. Scientific reports link *trans* fat (and saturated fat) with raising blood LDL ("bad") cholesterol levels, which increases your risk of coronary heart disease, a leading cause of death in the US.

Important: Health experts recommend that you *keep your intake of saturated fat, trans fat, and cholesterol as low as possible* as part of a nutritionally balanced diet.

Protein: A %DV is required to be listed if a claim is made for protein, such as "high in protein." Otherwise, unless the food is meant for use by infants and children under four years old, none is needed. Current scientific evidence indicates that protein intake is not a public health concern for adults and children over four years of age.

Sugars: No daily reference value has been established for sugars, because no recommendations have been made for the total amount to eat in a day. Keep in mind that the sugars listed on the Nutrition Facts label include naturally occurring sugars (like those in fruit and milk) as well as those added to a food or drink. Check the ingredient list for specifics on added sugars.

Take a look at the Nutrition Facts label for the two yogurt examples above. The plain yogurt on the left has 10 g of sugars, while the fruit yogurt on the right has 44 g of sugars in one serving.

Now look below at the ingredient lists for the two yogurts. Ingredients are listed in descending order of weight (from most to least). Note that no added sugars or sweeteners are in the list of ingredients for the plain yogurt, yet 10 g of sugars were listed on the Nutrition Facts label. This is because there are no added sugars in plain yogurt, only naturally occurring sugars (lactose in the milk).

Plain Yogurt—contains no added sugars:

INGREDIENTS: CULTURED PASTEURIZED GRADE A NONFAT MILK, WHEY PROTEIN CONCENTRATE, PECTIN, CARRAGEENAN.

Fruit Yogurt—contains added sugars:

INGREDIENTS: CULTURED GRADE A REDUCED FAT MILK, APPLES, HIGH FRUCTOSE CORN SYRUP, CINNAMON, NUTMEG, NATURAL FLAVORS, AND PECTIN. CONTAINS ACTIVE YOGURT AND L. ACIDOPHILUS CULTURES.

If you are concerned about your intake of sugars, make sure that added sugars are not listed as one of the first few ingredients. Other names for added sugars include: *corn syrup, high-fructose corn syrup, fruit juice concentrate, maltose, dextrose, sucrose, honey*, and *maple syrup.*

To *limit nutrients that have no %DV*, such as *trans* fat and sugars, compare the labels of similar products, and choose the food with the lowest amount.

Comparison Example:

Below are two kinds of milk: one is "reduced fat," the other is "nonfat." Each serving size is one cup. Which has more calories and more saturated fat? Which one has more calcium?

REDUCED FAT MILK   **NONFAT MILK**

2% Milk fat

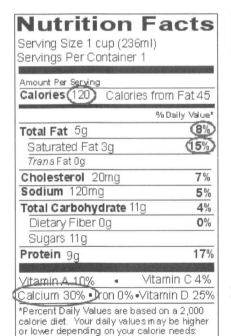

As you can see, they both have the same amount of calcium, but the nonfat milk has no saturated fat and has 40 calories less per serving than the reduced-fat milk.

Let's have a look at some of the optimal meal plans, anti-inflammatory diets, supplements, power foods, nutrient timings, and oxidative stress associated with nutrition.

Meal plans: Importance of meal combinations:

Certain foods are loaded with nutrients and fibers, while others are not: for example, green foods are much healthier than whole grains due to their higher fiber content and nutritional density.

When compared to two cups of broccoli, which has 9 g of fiber and 1,000 mg of potassium, two pieces of whole wheat bread yield a mere 4 g of fiber and around 140 mg of potassium.

It is considered that a typical American diet consists of only 15 g of fiber per day, which is 40–50 percent less than the recommended allowance of 25–30 g of fiber per day. The average American diet is typically low on greens.

Green vegetables can also serve as a good source of low-calorie meals; for example, ten cups of romaine lettuce contain only 160 calories; they yield 10 g of fiber and more than a 1,000 mg of potassium.

Due to the drastic differences in the nutrient values of foods and the way they are metabolized, the benefits of stacking nutrient-rich foods in an athlete's diet add up very quickly. For this reason it is important to study different food combinations and how to stack them for maximum athletic performance.

Rules to remember while creating your ideal meal plan:

The following principles hold true for nutrition regardless of whether you are a lightweight athlete or a heavyweight champion.

1. Pick starchy and fibrous carbohydrates instead of simple or refined carbohydrates.

Starchy carbohydrates usually have high amount of complex carbohydrates that take more time to break down. Simple and refined carbohydrates, on the other hand, are simple molecules that can be quickly absorbed into the blood.

By consuming starchy carbohydrates, you ensure that your body takes a longer time to digest the food; this ensures a steady supply of energy over a longer period of time. On the other hand, consuming a simple carbohydrate spikes up your blood-sugar levels and causes a quick burst of insulin into the bloodstream; such foods can be especially dangerous due to three major reasons:

1) Sudden bursts of insulin can increase the risk of diabetes.

2) Quick absorption of sugars causes a sudden spike in blood sugars followed by a sudden dip; this cause the person to feel irritable and hungry very fast.

Below is a list of healthy, starchy, and fibrous carbohydrates and fruits rich in dietary fibers. Try to add a larger portion of starch and fibrous carbohydrates to your meal plan; you may supplement your meals with a smaller serving of fruits rich in dietary fiber.

You can do a lot for your performance and health by eating foods that are not processed and are fresh, whole foods.

Carbohydrates list:

Starchy carbohydrates	Fibrous carbohydrates	Fruit rich in dietary fiber and simple carbohydrates
Green peas	Cauliflower	Apples
Carrots,	Mushrooms	Applesauce
Beet	Asparagus	Asian pears
White sweet corn, raw	Broccoli	Bananas
Sweet potato	Tomatoes	Pineapple
Potatoes	Green beans	Strawberries
Oatmeal	Cucumber	Blueberries
Lentils	Lettuce	Raspberries
Plantils	Spinach	Blackberries
Beans	Artichokes	Dates
Barley	Plantain	Figs
Yam	Turnip	Oranges
Brown rice, cream of rice	Okra	Peaches
Rye,	Brussels sprouts	Pears
Oat bran	Peas	Grapefruit
Whole grain bread (100%)	Squash	Prunes
Whole grain cereal (100%)	Zucchini	Raisins
Whole grain pasta (100%)	Salads	Tangerines
Other whole grains	Red and green pepper	
Legumes	Kale	

2. Divide your daily food intake into six equal proportions and spread them two to three hours apart throughout the day.

Why is this important?

Our human body has a very advanced metabolism that is sensitive to changes in blood sugar. Whenever we consume a meal, our blood sugars go up immediately, and these levels continue to decline constantly; it's important to realize that the gastric emptying time (time it takes for the food to empty out of the stomach) is two hours; therefore, if your stomach will become empty after two to three hours, it will lead to a drop in blood sugar; the gastric acids start pouring into your empty stomach, and you begin to feel the hunger pangs. The sheer craving can push you to grab a quick bite of some sugary snack just so you can get a quick fix of glucose, thus leading you to consume unhealthy foods very quickly.

If your body does not receive a fresh batch of nutrients, it goes into starvation mode and starts storing fat. This is especially bad, because our bodies start breaking the muscle tissue to maintain a constant flow of energy.

So here's rule number two: never allow your stomach to stay empty for more than two to three hours. Consuming small portions of food every two to three hours will ensure a healthy basic metabolic rate and encourage the body to burn fat for fuel.

3. Choose proteins over carbohydrates.

Protein is the most basic unit of a muscle, and you need to supply your body with plenty of protein, so that your body readily absorbs it at the peak of its anabolic demand, especially during and after your workout.

Protein also supports tissue regeneration and muscle repair on a daily basis. Protein is often ignored by endurance athletes; it is difficult to perform at optimal levels without adequate consumption of protein.

Protein has a high thermic effect: different types of foods require different amounts of energy to be broken down; this is known as the thermic effect of food.

The thermic effect of food starts as soon as the food enters the digestive tract, and it reaches its peak after about an hour of ingestion.

Proteins have a thermic effect of 30 percent, which implies that nearly 30 percent of the calories from proteins are used to digest the proteins. On the other hand, fats have a low thermic effect of 3 percent, which means that only 3 percent of the calories in fat are burned up for digestion.

Carbohydrate has a variable thermic effect: it fluctuates depending on source; the thermic effect is below 10 percent for pure sugars and in the 20–25 percent for starchy and fibrous foods.

Due to its high thermic effect and increased nitrogen demand in athletes, a high-protein diet can be very beneficial.

A recent study [1] on breakfasts revealed that consuming a high-protein breakfast along with a good dose of vitamin D and calcium helps in thermogenesis: higher rate of fat burning. It also reduced the overall calorie intake throughout the day. It has to be noted that the addition of vitamin D to protein is beneficial for maintaining a strict diet.

Meat, fish, and dairy are the only foods that provide vitamin D. You will likely want to supplement with vitamin D as well, because studies show that it is very difficult to fulfill your vitamin D needs from your diet alone.

As far as calcium is concerned, most of the protein sources are naturally high in calcium; men rarely need to take supplemental calcium; it should be noted that excessive intake of calcium can predispose to cardiac conduction abnormalities. Women may want to supplement their daily food intake with a small dose of calcium along with an adequate protein source and vitamin D.

Start your day with a healthy breakfast:

A good breakfast has the ability to keep you feeling fuller throughout the morning and reduces energy crashes and drowsiness.

The reduced levels of food intake and impulsive eating after high-protein meals are related to the release of ghrelin, a hunger hormone that increases your feelings of satiety and fullness.

Sources of protein

Protein can be obtained from almost all food sources. Let's discuss the different sources of protein:

1) Vegetable foods

2) Animal sources

3) Supplements

1) Vegetable sources of protein:

Vegetables are usually considered poor sources of protein, because almost no vegetable food provides all the essential amino acids necessary for muscle growth.

They are not a complete source of essential amino acids. Some sources such as soya beans have content of protein, but they do not provide all the essential amino acids.

Some health experts recommend combining different vegetable sources; for example, a mix of beans and rice can provide you with all the essential amino acids you need, but once you combine beans and rice, the quantity of food you consume increases, and the percentage of protein in rice and beans is much less when compared to animal sources of protein.

2) Animal sources of protein:

Animal protein contains almost all the essential amino acids in good quantities. Animal sources of protein include meat, eggs, and milk. The only issue with animal sources is the presence of large amounts of saturated fat, which have a lot of detrimental effects on the body.

The key here is to consume only lean cuts of meat and leave out saturated fat content.

Choose meats cut from the top round and lean cuts of sirloin and flank. The round is the rear leg of the cow or lamb. A frequently used muscle, the meat from this area is lean but tender. *Top round roast* refers to a lean and fairly tender cut as compared to the other cuts from the round. It has 10 percent of its calories from fat content.

Remove the skin in meat and avoid breaded forms of meat.

Eggs are an excellent source of protein; again, you want to leave out the saturated fat present in egg yolks and consume only the egg whites.

Below is a list of sources of lean animal protein:

chicken breast

fish and seafood

turkey breast

eggs (mostly whites—use limited yolks)

lean red meats (top round, lean sirloin, flank)

nonfat or low-fat dairy products

milk (low fat—1–2 percent) instead of whole milk products.

These foods need to be present in every meal, and you need to consume one meal every three hours in order to maintain a steady supply of protein.

3) Protein supplements:

Proteins are the building blocks of muscles; the body needs a continuous supply of protein to maintain its anabolic state. The body stays in an anabolic state for nearly forty-eight hours after exercise; this anabolic state has a high potential for producing lean muscle mass if an adequate supply of protein is maintained.

Following are recommendations for a safe, adequate protein intake (numbers are given for grams per pound of body weight, with an example for a 150-pound person):

- Sedentary person: 0.4 g/lb; 60 g

- Recreational exerciser, adult: 0.5–0.75 g/lb, 75–112 g

- Competitive athlete, adult: 0.6–0.9 g/lb, 90–135 g

- Growing teenage athlete: 0.8–0.9 g/lb, 120–135 g

- Dieting athlete, reduced calories: 0.8–0.9 g/lb, 120–135 g

- Maximum for all healthy athletes: 0.9 g/lb (2 g/kg)

For maximum benefits athletes are advised to divide their daily protein requirement into six meals and consume one meal every two to three hours.

Since this can be a time-consuming process, the athlete may opt for easier protein alternatives such as protein shakes and powder. The main advantage of consuming a protein supplement is convenience: all you need to do is consume the protein supplement mixed with milk or water and voila, all the essential amino acids are made available to your body instantly.

Suggested sample meal plans for high performance, muscle building, and fat burn:

- Divide your caloric intake into six portions.

- Your first two meals should contain one-third of the total calorie consumption.

- Your last two meals should ideally contain a lot of fibrous carbohydrates.

For breakfast:

Lean protein sources: egg whites (boiled, omelet, or scrambled); lean meats and fish; you may even include protein powder if you desire.

Starchy carbohydrate sources: whole-wheat bread and oatmeal.

Fat products (1–2 percent): skim milk, low-fat cheese, and natural peanut butter.

Fruits/juices: banana, apple, mango, and orange.

You want to make your first two meals from the choices you have above. These two meals should cover nearly one-third of your calorie intake.

Step1: Choose a source of lean protein plus one source of starchy carbohydrate.

Step 2: You may include simple carbohydrates such as fruits etc.

Step 3: You may add low-fat dairy products.

For other meals:

Your last four meals should contain two-thirds of your total calorie intake.

Step 1: Plan the amount of time you will dedicate to preparing your meals and how often you will prepare them (e.g., will you cook every session or every day or cook and store?).

Step 2: Choose a lean protein source for every dish you want to prepare.

Step 3: Choose a fibrous carbohydrate from the list for every dish you want to prepare.

Step 4: Add essential fats according to your diet plan; you may want to limit the fat intake, since the lean meats and other foods may have some fat content.

Step 5: Create a dish that is high on fibrous carbohydrates (two-thirds) and low on starchy carbohydrates (one-third).

Step 6: Create a recipe with only lean meat, high fibrous carbohydrate, very low complex carbs and essential fats; this will be your last two meals for the day to ensure maximum fat loss (carb tapering).

Step 7: Calculate the total calorie value, and check if it matches with your total calorie requirement.

Step 8: Allot a specific time for each meal, and never skip a meal.

If you are the type who enjoys cooking and likes to cook every meal, then you can have a lot of variety, and, on the other hand, if you are the busy type with no time for leisurely cooking, then you can cook your meals and store them.

Depending on the place you live and the kind of ethnic background you have, you may have your own cooking style, but as long as you follow the basic laws, you will enjoy high performance and experience quicker recovery after a training session.

How to fight inflammation:

Dr. David Seaman is one of the leading authorities on anti-inflammatory diets; he came up with the concept of deflame diet and advised that certain foods can be used as medicine to heal the body.

While in clinical practice in the mid 1980s, he became aware of the developing research that linked nutrition to the inflammatory process and noticed that appropriate dietary changes could significantly improve various musculoskeletal and visceral conditions; he wrote the foundational book on anti-inflammation, *Clinical Nutrition for Pain, Inflammation and Tissue Healing*, nearly ten years ago.

Since then Dr. Seaman has always been well ahead of the curve on how different foods can up- or down-regulate the metabolic reactions that promote or suppress inflammation.

The next section discusses various components of an effective anti-inflammatory diet. More tips, resources, and "deflaming" guidelines can be found on his website, www.deflame.com.

Pro-inflammatory foods:

Many different foods, such as sugar, trans fats, processed foods, and foods cooked at very high temperatures can lead to internal inflammation, which can harm the body at a fundamental level and slow down recovery.

Diseases associated with this condition include constant headaches, arthritis, fibromyalgia, chronic fatigue syndrome, sinusitis, allergies, acne, asthma, chronic pain, dysmenorrhea, cancer, heart disease, osteoporosis, multiple sclerosis, Parkinson's disease, Alzheimer's disease, hypertension, and depression.

Here's a list of pro-inflammatory foods that should be avoided

1. Simple, processed, and refined carbohydrates:

- white and whole-wheat breads
- sugars and sugary snacks
- sugar drinks, including fruit juices that contain added sugars
- canned foods with lots of sodium
- white breads and pastas made with refined white flour
- high-fat convenience foods
- frozen dinners
- packaged cakes and cookies, including bagels, breads, rolls, and other baked goods
- boxed meal mixes
- sugary breakfast cereals
- corn syrup
- popcorn
- crackers
- croissants
- doughnuts
- egg rolls
- fast food
- french fries
- fruit juice—choose the fruit instead
- fried foods
- flour
- granola
- hard cheese (except for feta and grating cheeses, such as Romano and Parmesan)
- honey
- hot dogs
- ice cream, frozen yogurt, Italian ices

• potatoes	• jams, jellies, and preserves
• pudding	• margarine
• relish	• molasses
• rice	• muffins
• sherbet	• noodles
• shortening	• pancakes
• snack foods, including potato chips, pretzels, corn chips, and rice and corn cakes	• waffles
	• tortillas
• tacos	

2. Common cooking oils:

A few cooking oils are known to promote inflammation, since they are made from cheap ingredients that are not healthy: these include soy, sunflower, corn, cottonseed, safflower, peanut, and soybean oil, and foods derived from these oils, including mayonnaise, tartar sauce, margarine, salad dressings, and packaged foods.

3. Dairy:

Milk can very often serve as a trigger for inflammation, stomach problems, skin rashes, hives, and even breathing difficulties.

4. Fresh or frozen fish:

A recent study published in the *Journal of the American Diet Association*[2] revealed that farmed-raised tilapia, catfish, and bronzini had unacceptable omega-6 to omega-3 ratios, while all other fish had appropriate ratios.

Foods that are anti-inflammatory:

1. *Unsaturated fats* have a wide range of health benefits; it has been noted that replacing saturated fats with unsaturated fats helps lower the levels of bad cholesterol (LDL) in the blood.

There are two types of unsaturated fats: monounsaturated and polyunsaturated.

A fat molecule is monounsaturated if it contains one double bond, and polyunsaturated if it contains more than one double bond.

Monounsaturated fat: Studies show that eating foods rich in monounsaturated fats (MUFAs) improves blood levels of good cholesterol (HDL), which can in turn decreases symptoms of inflammation in the body. Research also shows that MUFAs may benefit insulin levels and blood-sugar control, which can be especially helpful in preventing Type 2 diabetes.

Sources of MUFA: Olive oil contains about 75 percent monounsaturated fat, and tea-seed oil contains over 80 percent monounsaturated fat. Canola oil and cashews contain about 58 percent monounsaturated fat. Other sources include macadamia nuts; grape-seed, groundnut (peanut oil), sesame, corn, and avocado oil; as well as popcorn, cereal, oatmeal, and tea-oil *Camellia*.

Recommended sources of monounsaturated fat

- avocados

- cashews

- peanuts

- pecans

- natural peanut butter

- olives

- olive oil

Polyunsaturated fat: This type of fat improves good cholesterol (HDL) levels in blood, which can decrease your risk of heart disease and improve cardiovascular function and overall stamina. PUFAs also help decrease the risk of Type 2 diabetes.

PUFAs are found in sesame oil.

The United States Food and Drug Administration (USFDA) recommends that the amount of unsaturated fat consumption should not exceed 30 percent of one's daily caloric intake (or 67 grams, given a 2,000-calorie diet).

2. Essential fatty acids (EFAs) and their benefits: EFAs are fatty acids that humans and other animals must ingest, because the body requires them for good health.

Only two EFAs are recommended for human consumption: alpha-linolenic acid (an omega-3 fatty acid) and linoleic acid (an omega-6 fatty acid).

Essential fatty acids have a wide range of benefits: they are known to improve insulin sensitivity, they help in better transport of oxygen, and produce higher quality of energy; they have anti-oxidant and anti-aging properties, and they help in improving the texture and smoothness of skin.

EFAs also help reduce signs of moodiness and depression by reducing the levels of cortisol (stress hormones) in the body. In terms of metabolism, essential fatty acids increase the metabolic rate and burn down excess fat.

Many research studies [38] have shown that omega 3 fatty acids have many anti-inflammatory and immune modulating effects.

The two most common types of components that make up most omega 3 fatty acid supplements are docosahexaenoic acid (DHA) and eicosapentaenoic acid (EPA).

Omega-3 fatty acid EPA is known to be a direct precursor for the anti-inflammatory prostaglandins E1 and E3, and DHA plays a major role in maintaining the structural integrity of neuronal membranes. DHA is also responsible for brain and visual development.

Both EPA and DHA can be consumed in the form of fish-oil capsules. Other sources of EPA and DHA are flaxseed, flaxseed oil, fish, and krill oils; these oils should be kept refrigerated. Whole flaxseeds need to be ground within 24 hours prior to use; this helps the ingredients to stay active. Flaxseeds are also available in ground form in a special Mylar package, so the components in the flaxseeds stay active.

While buying omega-3 fatty acid supplements, always choose certified companies that make products that are free of heavy metals such as mercury, lead, and cadmium.

Food sources that contain both omega-3 and omega-6 fatty acids:

- fatty fish: Salmon contains anti-inflammatory omega-3s and is known to help in healing. Try and incorporate oily fish into your diet twice weekly. If you don't like fish, try a high quality fish supplement.

- shellfish

- flaxseed (linseed)

- hemp oil, soya oil, canola (grapeseed) oil

- chia seeds, pumpkin seeds, sunflower seeds

- leafy vegetables

- walnuts

3. Flaxseed oil:

- It is often believed that fish oil and fish products are the best sources of EFAs; however, flaxseed oil is known to contain at least twice the amount of omega-3 fatty acids as seen in fish.

- Many experts recommend intake of one tablespoon of flaxseed oil a day to meet the daily requirement of EFAs, and the maximum limit can be up to five tablespoons per day.

- However, it should be noted that flaxseed oil contains low amounts of omega-6 fatty acids, and the ratio of omega-3 fatty acids to omega-6 fatty acids is 4:1.

- Some experts recommend making your own your own "oil blend" by mixing three parts flaxseed with one part sunflower oil.

4. Extra virgin olive oil:

Olive oil contains a strong dose of fats that fight inflammation; the oil is known to reduce risks of arthritis and asthma, and it is known to benefit the cardiovascular system.

5. Kelp:

Kelp has traditionally been known for its cancer-fighting properties; it is also known for its strong anti-inflammatory properties, high fiber content, and antioxidant properties. Kelp is a brown-algae extract: kombu, wakame, and arame are good sources.

6. Cruciferous vegetables:

These vegetables are known to be rich in antioxidants; cruciferous vegetables include brussels sprouts, broccoli, kale, and cauliflower.

These vegetables can detoxify the body and eliminate any harmful compounds.

7. Blueberries:

Blueberries are known to have several benefits, which include anti-inflammatory, neuro-protective, and anti-cancer properties. It is important to choose organic blueberries to avoid contamination with pesticides.

8. Turmeric:

Turmeric is known for its anti-inflammatory properties. Turmeric is considered as an Asian spice and can be used in the preparation of curries.

9. Vitamin-C-rich foods:

Vitamin C stimulates the production of white blood cells and antibodies to fight off infection. Many fruits and vegetables are good sources of vitamin C—the best being citrus fruits, kiwi fruit, strawberries, and melons. Green vegetables such as kale, asparagus, broccoli, beans, and peas are also rich in vitamin C, so be sure to include plenty of fruit and vegetables in your diet to give your immune system the support it needs.

10. Garlic and onions:

Garlic and onions not only flavor the food you eat, they also help the immune system by stimulating the production of infection-busting white blood cells.

Garlic can also help regulate glucose and help reduce inflammation. As an added bonus, garlic helps keep your heart healthy by stopping blood platelets from sticking together, thus keeping blood vessels clear to promote good circulation.

11. Green Tea:

Green tea contains several anti-inflammatory flavonoids that may even help reduce the risks of certain cancers.

12. Sweet Potato:

Sweet potatoes are known to have anti-inflammatory properties. They are also great sources of beta-carotene, manganese, fiber, and vitamins C and B6.

13. Cherries:

Cherries have several benefits; they promote better sleep, nutrition, and aid better circulation. Tart cherries are a natural source of melatonin; consuming a tart cherry supplement prior to sleep can lower your body temperature and help you sleep better.

Sweet cherries have high potassium content and serve as a natural anti-hypertensive (blood-pressure-lowering agent); they help in achieving fluid balance in the body. Cherries also contain high levels of anthocyanins, which act as antioxidants and help promote recovery. To add to all the list of benefits above, cherries are rich in vitamins A, C, and E: they contain nineteen times more betacarotenes than blueberries. Due to their powerful anti-inflammatory benefits, cherries are said to reduce pain and joint soreness for runners and athletes after workouts.

14. Elderberries:

Elderberries are fruits born by the elder tree, and they play an important role in helping raise immunity levels and fighting inflammation. Elderberries are rich in natural substances known as flavonoids; these substances help in fighting off inflammation and boosting immunity. Research studies [39] have shown that elderberry reduces flu symptoms such as fever, sore throat, fatigue, body aches, and headache if started within twenty-four to forty-eight hours after the symptoms begin.

Elderberry also helps fight off bronchitis and bacterial sinus infections.

Dosage: currently there are no established guidelines or recommended dosages for elderberry consumption—this supplement may be taken in doses (usually one tablespoon of elderberry syrup extract four times a day) recommended by the manufacturer.

Avoid eating any foods or consuming any fruit drinks manufactured from raw elderberry, since it is known to cause side effects; the preferred substance for consumption is elderberry syrup extract, and it should be taken only when the athlete experiences signs/symptoms of flu, nasal allergies, sinusitis, or bronchitis.

How to choose at the supermarket:

Pick your food wisely:

- **Choose grass-fed sources of meat:** A list of grass-fed animal products can be found at www.eatwild.com; this is important, because most of the industry-fed animals are unnaturally fat and can be unhealthy, since they contain high levels of saturated fats and pro-inflammatory omega-6 fatty acids.

  If you are unable to use grass-fed animal products, then choose lean cuts of meat from a trusted supermarket.

- **Omega-3 eggs:** Many supermarkets carry eggs that are rich in omega-3 and have anti-inflammatory properties.

- These products include:

1) Christopher Eggs (600 mg omega-3 per egg yolk),

2) 4-Grain Vegetarian Omega-3 Eggs (300 mg omega-3 per yolk),

3) Sparboe Farms Omega-3 Eggs (250 mg omega3 per yolk),

4) Eggland's Best (110 mg omega-3 per yolk).

- **Choice of butter:** Butter can be considered healthy when it comes from grass-fed cows. Some supermarkets carry organic butter (made from grass-fed cows).

- **Choice of salad dressings:** Extra virgin olive oil, balsamic vinegar (or lemon juice), mustard if you like, and spices (Greek, Italian, ginger, dill, oregano, etc.; whatever suits your taste). When eating in a restaurant, use dressings sparingly, as most are made with soybean oil or worse, and most are rich in sugar.

- **Choice of alcohol:** Red wine contains resveratrol and other antioxidants that are good for heart function. Choose stout beer if you want to drink beer.

- **Spices:** Spices can boost immunity indirectly. By stimulating digestive enzymes, they improve your body's ability to extract nutrients from foods. They benefit immunity directly through their antioxidant value. In fact, they are really "super foods." Here's a spice mixture for enhancing immunity. Grind the mixture below:

  - 3 parts turmeric

  - 3 parts ground cumin

  - 3 parts ground coriander

- 1 part ground fennel

- 1 part powdered ginger

- 1 part ground black pepper

- 1/4 part ground cinnamon

- 1/4 part ground cardamom

- 1 part chili powder/paprika

Mix all the powdered spices well and store in an airtight container in a cool place away from direct sun. Some people will want to omit the fennel and/or the cardamom.

Use this mixture to add taste to your food; add a little bit to your cooking food in the last stage. This can work with grains, legumes, vegetables, and even meats and fish.

Consume more fruits and vegetables: Eat fruits raw and vegetables raw or lightly cooked. Red and sweet potatoes are acceptable as long as they are consumed with a protein, such as eggs, fish, meat, or fowl.

Special note—cottonseed oil: In his book *Eight Weeks to Optimum Health,* Dr. Weil recommends his readers to go through their pantry shelves and throw out anything made with cottonseed oil. Cottonseed oil contains high levels of saturated fat and is too low in monounsaturated fat. Cottonseed oil is also known to contain many natural toxins and unacceptably high levels of pesticide residues (cotton is not classified as a food crop, and farmers use many agrichemicals when growing it).

It is important to note that manufacturers like cottonseed oils because they are cheap; certain packaged foods contain cottonseed oil in them;

therefore, make sure you read the ingredient labels of products and avoid foods with cottonseed oil.

Supplements:

The supplements listed below can decrease inflammation (local and global) and free-radical formation.

A. **Omega-3 fatty acid**—1,000–4,000mg: Benefits and sources of omega-3 fatty acids are discussed in the previous section. For athletes I like a product made by Douglas Labs that has 600 mg EPA and 400 mg of DHA with 1,000 mg of vitamin D3, from small fish such as anchovies or sardines. These oils are ultra-pure and either supercritical-CO2-extracted or molecularly distilled to remove heavy metals including arsenic, cadmium, lead, mercury, dioxins, and PCB.

B. **CoQ10**—50 mg–200 mg: Coenzyme Q10 is present in every cell of the body; it is also known as ubiquinone, which comes from the word *ubiquitous*, because it is found everywhere in the body.

Coenzyme Q10 helps in the production of ATP (energy) in the mitochondria of the cell.

The cells in our body break down sugars, proteins, and fats to create energy. CoQ10 is essential for this reaction; our body is able to produce CoQ10 naturally, but when the body suffers oxidative damage and inflammatory damage, CoQ10 is the first enzyme to be depleted.

Coenzyme Q10 is known to have antioxidant properties and plays a major role in cardiovascular health and physical energy.

Studies have shown that patients who were suffering from high cholesterol and were placed on statin drugs could prevent the associated muscle damage by consuming 10 to 50 mg of CoQ10 daily.

Recommended dosage for CoQ10:

CoQ10 is available in a wide variety of doses ranging from 10 mg to 300 mg; however, the dose of 50–200 mg is adequate for daily use, unless a higher dose is recommended for medical conditions.

Benefits of CoQ10:

Anti-inflammatory effect: it's been found that co-supplementation with vitamin E and coenzyme Q10 reduces circulating markers of inflammation indicated by the CRP concentration in healthy adult baboons. [3]

Other benefits include reduced levels of bad cholesterol, protection against diabetes and high blood sugar, better gum health, and reduced levels of fatigue.

Side effects: Very high doses of CoQ10 (more than 300 mg) can lead to tiredness, increased sleep, or cause insomnia.

C. Phytosterols:

What are phytosterols?

Phytosterols are cholesterol-like molecules found in plants; they are commonly known as plant sterols. Whereas animal cholesterols are considered unhealthy, plant sterols are considered to be good for the human body; this is because phytosterols are not absorbed very well by the intestine, and as a result they do not enter the blood stream.

Phytosterols are good because they slow down the absorption of regular cholesterol from the diet.

Many studies have been conducted to examine the effect of phytosterols on lowering blood cholesterol. It's been found that addition of up to 2 g of phytosterols per day can produce a 10 percent reduction of low-density-like proteins (bad cholesterol) within two weeks. [4]

The Food and Drug Administration now allows phytosterol containing products to be labeled as "heart healthy."

Eating fruits and vegetables can provide you with a good source of phytosterols; additionally you may check food labels to select foods that contain phytosterols, or you may choose to add a supplement containing phytosterols to your diet. Two tablets of Centrum Cardio provide 800 mg of phytosterols.

As always, it is important to monitor how you feel after taking supplements, because the effects of supplements are different on different individuals. Adding a supplement to your daily regimen can provide a wide range of benefits such as improved energy, better stamina, and better recovery; however, when you're picking a natural supplement, it is important to monitor for side effects such as muscle and joint pain, tiredness, weakness, fatigue, and mood and sleep patterns for the first two weeks, before making the supplement a permanent part of your daily regimen.

D. Spices: Turmeric, ginger, cinnamon—use to season your food (discussed in the previous section).

E. Magnesium, 200–1,000 mg: Discussed in the previous section.

F. Multivitamins: Vitamins and minerals are micronutrients required to ensure the proper functioning of your metabolism.

Many of these nutrients are present in a well-balanced diet; however, the absence of a particular vitamin due to a restricted diet or poor quality of food may affect the athlete's performance and recovery.

For this reason adding a multivitamin, multi-mineral pill can serve as an insurance against poor body metabolism and poor performance.

Special note:

Vitamin B has been linked to high performance in athletes. Vitamin B includes thiamin, riboflavin, and vitamins B-6, B-12, and folate.

Studies conducted by the Oregon State University demonstrated that athletes who are deficient in B vitamins have a reduced capacity for high-intensity exercise, and the recovery rate for damaged muscles is much lower when compared to their competitors who consumed diets rich in vitamin B.

It's been found that exercise can increase the athlete's requirement for riboflavin and vitamin B6; exercise also increases the production of free radicals and subsequent cellular damage.

Studies published in *International Journal of Sport Nutrition and Exercise Metabolism* reveal that even small levels of vitamin B deficiency can affect performance and recovery. Vitamin B consumption becomes extremely important in athletes who follow restricted diet plans; therefore, it is important to consume a supplement containing vitamin B.

Consumption of *vitamin C* is known to boost immunity; whenever possible vitamin C should be consumed in its purest form, which is ascorbic acid powder of pharmaceutical grade. Ascorbic acid (vitamin C) powder tastes a bit like diluted table salt; it can be mixed with a cup of water and consumed three to four times per day.

Caution: It is important to note that some athletes do not tolerate vitamin C very well and may experience diarrhea after a heavy dose of vitamin C; in such cases smaller divided doses of vitamin C are recommended.

The good news is that vitamins B and C are water-soluble, hence any excess of vitamins B and C are readily flushed out through urine.

Below is a list of essential vitamins, [5] their recommended daily allowance, and foods that are rich in these vitamins.

Vitamin	Men	Women	Sources
A	0.7 mg	0.6 mg	cheese, eggs, oily fish such as mackerel, milk, fortified low-fat spreads, yogurt
B6	1.4 mg	1.2 mg	pork, chicken, turkey, cod, bread, whole cereals such as oatmeal, wheat germ and rice, eggs, vegetables, soya beans, peanuts, milk, potatoes, some fortified breakfast cereals
B12	0.0015 mg	0.0015 mg	meat, salmon, cod, milk, cheese, eggs, yeast extract, some fortified breakfast cereals
B3 (niacin)	17 mg	13 mg	meat, fish, wheat flour, maize flour, eggs, milk
Pantothenic acid	200 mg	200 mg	chicken, beef, potatoes, porridge, tomatoes, kidney, eggs, broccoli, whole grains, such as brown rice and whole-meal bread
B2 (riboflavin)	1.3 mg	1.1 mg	milk, eggs, fortified breakfast cereals, rice, mushrooms
B1 (thiamin)	1 mg	0.8 mg	pork, vegetables, milk, cheese, peas, fresh and dried fruit, eggs, whole-grain breads
Folic Acid	0.2 mg	0.2 mg	broccoli, brussels sprouts, asparagus, peas, chickpeas, brown rice
C	40 mg	40 mg	peppers, broccoli, brussels sprouts, sweet potatoes, oranges, kiwi fruit
D	0.025 mg	0.025 mg	oily fish such as salmon and sardines, eggs, fortified fat spreads, fortified breakfast cereals, powdered milk
E	4 mg	3 mg	nuts and seeds, wheat germ found in cereals and cereal products
K	0.001 mg	0.001 mg	green and leafy vegetables such as broccoli and spinach, vegetable oils, cereals

G. Quercetin: Many plants and foods contain the pigment quercetin.

Sources of quercetin: red wine, apples, Gingko biloba, berries, green tea, and onion.

Quercetin is known to contain medicinal properties. Quercetin has a positive effect on the heart and blood vessels due to its antioxidant and anti-inflammatory properties.

It has been widely included in natural supplements to reduce prostate inflammation. To date it's been found that quercetin is can help in the treatment of inflammation, asthma, viral infections, gout, chronic fatigue syndrome, and also can help in preventing cancer.

Quercetin is especially useful for sports athletes, because research studies [6, 7] have revealed that consuming 500 mg of quercetin twice daily for three weeks before participating in intense cycling competitions reduces the number of upper-respiratory infections during and after the period of heavy exercise. It is also known to improve exercise endurance.

Side effects: Quercetin has shown no significant side effects when a dose of 500 mg is consumed twice daily for twelve weeks. Long-term studies (longer than three months) have not been carried out so far; however, no significant side effects have been reported by long-term users of quercetin.

Very high doses of quercetin may cause tingling sensation in the limbs and headache.

Special note: Quercetin should not be taken along with antibiotics, since they may interact with the antibiotics and reduce their efficacy.

F. Resveratrol:

Resveratrol belongs to the group of polyphenols, and it occurs as a natural compound in many plants. Resveratrol has gained popularity due to its antioxidant properties and its protective capability against diseases such as cancer, inflammatory damage, and heart disease.

Sources of resveratrol:

Resveratrol can be found in peanuts, berries, and, most importantly, in red grape skins.

Resveratrol supplements sold in the market are manufactured from Chinese and Japanese knotweed plants (*Polygonum cuspidatum*), followed by supplements that contain resveratrol extracted from red grape and red wine extracts, which are typically more expensive.

Benefits of resveratrol [8, 9]:

Anti-inflammatory nature: Resveratrol helps in fighting off inflammation in the body; it prevents the oxidation of LDL and reduces the stickiness of platelets.

Anti-cancer properties: Resveratrol plays a major role in apoptosis (a scientific term used to describe cancer cell death) and limits the spread of cancer cells.

Long-term use of resveratrol has been shown to be neuro-protective and helps in the prevention of Alzheimer's disease.

Many commercial institutes have claimed that resveratrol has anti-aging properties; however, this claim is yet to be backed by solid clinical studies.

Side-effects and precautions:

Since resveratrol has certain blood-thinning properties, it should be avoided in patients receiving blood thinners such as warfarin and non-steroidal anti-inflammatory medications such as aspirin and ibuprofen, due to increased risk for bleeding.

H. Glutathione:

Glutathione is a small molecule found in every cell of the body; it is a natural antioxidant, since it is found within every cell.

The most commonly known antioxidants are vitamins C and E; however, due to its position within the cell, glutathione can act as a more effective antioxidant, thus neutralizing the damage caused by free radicals.

Benefits of glutathione:

Glutathione helps the liver excrete chemicals, drugs, and pollutants that can harm the body. Glutathione is known to have antioxidant properties; it is used in the treatment of diseases that weaken the immune system, preventing aging, memory loss, and chronic fatigue syndrome.

Glutathione helps in maintaining intracellular health; studies have revealed that glutathione helps in recovery from illness [10] and training. [11]

Sources of glutathione:

Glutathione content is high in fresh fruit, vegetables, and fresh meats. A balanced diet may contain adequate levels of glutathione required by the body; however, athletes on restricted diets are often short on glutathione and can benefit from supplementation (250–500 mg per day).

F. Potassium:

Potassium is not just a mineral; it also serves as an electrolyte and helps in conduction of electrical signals across skeletal muscles and various tissues of the body. It is stored along with glycogen and helps in transporting glucose into muscle cells.

Potassium facilitates proper skeletal muscle movement, sodium regulation, and cell/organ function. An athlete may require more amounts of potassium than a regular person due to electrolyte loss during exercise.

It is very vital to learn how to identify the symptoms of low potassium in the body. Studies (Knochel 1978 and 1982) have revealed that potassium deficiency can be can be responsible for muscle injury and can be induced by a variety of mechanisms. Loss of potassium is amplified during training sessions in hot climates.

Symptoms of potassium deficiency/low potassium levels:

- generalized muscle weakness
- slower reflexes in the body
- muscle cramps
- irregular heart rate
- stomach disturbance

Causes of low potassium:

The most common cause of low potassium in athletes is excessive loss of potassium via sweat and usage of potassium for muscle movement during sport.

Sources of potassium:

According to the University of Illinois, athletes need not consume supplement pills to regulate potassium levels; instead a good supply of potassium can be availed from fresh fruits. Many fruits such as bananas and oranges contain high levels of potassium. Potassium is also present in high levels in baked potato.

Other good sources of potassium include the following:

• beet greens	• avocados
• white beans	• tomatoes
• yogurt	• lima beans
• flounder	• salmon
• cod	• chicken
• citrus juices	• cantaloupes

It is important to note that while potassium replenishment is important, excessive intake of potassium can lead to hyperkalemia and affect heart function due to altered electrical conductivity in heart muscle.

A quick analysis of potassium can be obtained by doing a biochemical study of blood electrolytes.

We do see that some endurance athletes, among others, need to supplement with potassium, and this may be in the form of sports drinks or supplements. The key is to have your blood tested for key nutrients such as potassium, magnesium, and vitamin D to find out if you are in need.

Practical tips:

- Changes in body weight: fluid loss and electrolyte loss can often be detected by studying the body weight before and after training sessions.

- By checking your weight every morning after urinating, you can understand whether you are consuming excess fluids or if there is a loss of electrolytes. Fluid/electrolyte loss or gain often manifests with a change in more than 0.5 kg in one day; this is drastically different from gradual weight gain or weight loss noticed in training programs.

- Restwise: Restwise revolutionizes the process of preparing your body for endurance performance. It uses research-based markers that relate to recovery and overtraining, determines their relative importance, and generates a meaningful calculation that tells an athlete how prepared his or her body is for hard training. This tool will be discussed in detail in future sections.

- Another way to look for excessive fluid loss is by observing the color of urine each morning after urinating. If the color of urine is darker than usual, then it indicates that you are probably dehydrated and need to consume more fluids during the day.

- Prior to training: drinking fruit juice or an electrolyte solution two hours prior to the exercise/training session can help in preventing dehydration.

- During heightened periods of training, it is important to consume sports drinks throughout the day.

Immune support:

1. Vitamin D:

Vitamin D may be readily found in dietary sources such as eggs, milk, fish, and cod liver oil. Exposure to sunlight also increases the production vitamin D; it's been found that just ten to fifteen minutes of exposure to sunlight can boost the production vitamin D.

The most important function of vitamin D is to help in the metabolism of phosphorus and calcium. Vitamin D helps in the formation of strong bones, because it helps in the absorption of calcium into the bone matrix.

Lack of vitamin D may lead to muscle weakness, increased appetite, and osteomalacia (bone disorder). Regular supplementation with vitamin D has also proven to be effective in raising levels of immunity and reducing levels of depression.

Recommended dosage:

The guidelines, released by the Institute of Medicine (IOM) call for increased rates of RDA for vitamin D: the new recommended daily allowance (RDA), as set in 2010, is based on age, as follows:

600 IU daily for those one to seventy years of age

800 IU daily for those seventy-one years and older

600 IU daily for pregnant and lactating women

The IOM further recommended that serum 25(OH)D levels of 20 mg/mL (= 50 nmol/L) is adequate, and levels greater than 50 ng/mL (= 125 nmol/L) could have potential adverse effects.

2. Vitamin C: Vitamin C can play a major role in boosting immunity. Its role is discussed in the previous section.

3. Zinc: Zinc is commonly called an essential trace element, because minute quantities of this mineral are essential for optimal health.

Zinc plays an important role in strengthening the immune system, thereby helping us fight signs of flu, common cold, and other recurrent infections.

Zinc is important for athletic performance, because it helps in tissue repair and recovery after exercise. Zinc also helps in the conversion of food to fuel. Athletes typically have lower levels of zinc due to increased levels of usage. Zinc depletion during exercise is considered to be one of the major factors for compromised immunity after extended periods of exercise. [13]

Athletes who train without breaks often run a serious risk of losing zinc very quickly. Studies conducted on cyclists [14] with varying levels of training intensity reveal different levels of zinc depletion associated with different intensity of activity; athletes who participated in heavy training over a period of two months lost more zinc than athletes who trained at a moderate level for two to three weeks.

One of the reasons for this phenomenon could be an altered zinc metabolism along with increased levels of zinc depletion. Decreased levels of zinc lead to decreased levels of endurance in sports and causes fatigue.

The recommended dose of zinc is between 30 and 60 mg per day. [15] The most tolerated doses of zinc are zinc picolinate or monomethionate. [16]

4. Glutamine:

Glutamine provides massive benefits for sports athletes. Glutamine helps in the increase of total number of lymphocytes and macrophages, thereby increasing the immunity of the athlete.

Research studies [17] reveal that these immune cells show low levels of activity when a person is low on glutamine.

Prolonged levels of exercise are also known to lower levels of glutamine. Glutamine supplementation reduces the risk of infections after a long term of stressful exercise. [18]

A recent study analyzed the effect of glutamine supplementation of two hundred runners and rowers; these athletes were given a supplementation of 2,000 mg of placebo or glutamine two hours after exercise.

During the seven day follow-up, it was found that 81 percent of the subjects who consumed the Glutamine supplement remained disease free, whereas only 49 percent of the individuals in the placebo group remained disease-free. [19] This clearly shows that glutamine can increase immunity in athletes.

Glutamine also prevents muscle breakdown after an exercise period.

Recommended dosage: a supplementation of 2 g of glutamine given following exercise can boost the immunity and recovery rate in athletes.

This is all the more important for athletes who undertake heavy loads of training and exercise prior to a competition. Adequate supplementation in athletes can help in quicker recovery, better immunity, lower infection rates, and better performance.

5. Probiotics:

Probiotics are good bacteria that help the digestive system and improve gut metabolism; the Food and Agriculture Organization of the United Nations (FAO) defines them as "live microorganisms, which, when administered in adequate amounts, confer a health benefit on the host."

Probiotics are important for athletes, because strenuous exercise, dieting, and environmental changes can upset the balance of good bacteria in the gut.

Numerous health benefits have been attributed to probiotics, including improvement of gastrointestinal tract function and diseases, immune function, hyperlipidemia, hypertension, and allergic conditions. [22]

Research studies [20] conducted by A.J Cox et al. (2007) revealed that probiotic supplements help reduce the length of infections and number of infections suffered by long-distance runners.

The study conducted by the Australian Institute of Sport in Canberra followed training and recovery patterns in twenty top long-distance runners during the intensive winter training program for a period of four months; all twenty athletes received either a probiotic supplement with *Lactobacillus fermentum* or a placebo containing no active ingredients.

During the four-month follow-up, the group that was on a placebo complained of experiencing symptoms of cold and respiratory symptoms for a total of seventy-two days, whereas the group that was on probiotic supplementation experienced only thirty days of sickness.

Further lab tests revealed that the athletes who had consumed probiotic supplements had doubled levels of interferon gamma (a molecule that helps in improving immunity).

Such improved resistance to common illnesses can serve as an important benefit for athletes taking part in strenuous sports.

Studies revealed that athletes who consumed probiotics reported quicker rates of recovery after strenuous exercise; other positive benefits include lesser incidence of stomach and intestinal upset.

Probiotics also proved effective in reducing the incidence of Epstein Barr virus (EBV), which causes chronic fatigue syndrome. The saliva samples obtained from eight athletes participating in strenuous exercise before and after one month of acidophilus (probiotic) supplementation showed an 80 percent reduction in EBV infection; prior to the start of acidophilus supplementation, five athletes suffered from EBV infection, whereas only one athlete tested positive for EBV infection (chronic fatigue syndrome) after one month of supplementation. The most significant change before and after the supplementation was the improvement of CD4 function (white blood cell), which helped in immune function.

Sources of probiotics:

Probiotics can be found in fermented food products such as yogurt, sauerkraut, kefir, cabbage kimchee, and soybean-based miso and natto. Additionally many sports nutrition stores carry cost-effective priobiotic supplements.

6. Echinacea

Echinacea is a floral extract available in many health food stores that sell herbal supplements. Echinacea earned its reputation as herb with the ability to shorten the duration of cold and flu if consumed at the onset of symptoms.

Researchers [23] studied the effects of echinacea, magnesium, and placebo from twenty-eight days prior to a triathlon event to forty-four hours after finishing the race.

The results of the research were significant; usually strenuous periods of exercise produces inflammatory responses within the body, and this is evidenced by the raised levels of natural killer (NK) cells, total T lymphocyte count, and interleukin counts.

As expected, the athletes in the magnesium and placebo group showed increase in levels of these inflammatory factors, but the group that was supplemented with echinacea showed a reduction in the levels of inflammatory markers. Furthermore, thirteen athletes in the magnesium group developed signs of cold or flu and had to miss thirteen days of training; the athletes in the placebo group missed a total of twenty-four days of training, whereas the athletes in the echinacea group did not miss a single day of training.

This study supports the long-held views about echinacea being a health-restoring agent if consumed during the early stages of flu or cold.

Recommended doses for echinacea:

Unlike most supplements, echinacea should not be consumed every day. The maximum consecutive use is about ten to fourteen days. For illness, it's best to take echinacea during the first signs of a cold or flu coming on.

- Dried form: can be used to make tea—1–2 grams of dried root can be used for this purpose.

- Liquid extract: 2–3 ml

- Powdered extract containing 4 percent phenolics: 300 mg may be used to boost immunity for 1–2 weeks.

7. **Osillococcinum** is known to provide temporary relief from symptoms of flu, which include headache, body aches, low energy, fever, and chills. It serves as a handy home remedy for flulike symptoms. Although the research is very limited and anecdotal, this supplement may offer some help in fighting flu symptoms.

8. Airborne supplements have provided symptomatic relief in athletes suffering from flulike symptoms; however, the efficacy of these supplements has not been proven.

9. Zicam supplements have provided symptomatic relief in athletes suffering from cold and allergy symptoms; however, the efficacy of these supplements has not been proven.

* **Don't-get-sick pack**: echinacea, oscillococcinum, Airborne, and Zicam

Injury Care:

A. Glucosamine/MSM blend: The methylsulfonylmethane (MSM)/ glucosamine blend is known to reduce joint pain and inflammation. MSM is a natural sulfur compound found in the tissues and fluids or all living organisms.

Glucosamine is an amino sugar; however, it is not used as a source of energy; instead it gets incorporated into the structure of tissues and helps in the formation of nails, tendons, skin, eyes, bones, and heart valves; it also helps in the production of mucous secretion of the digestive, respiratory, and urinary tracts.

MSM/glucosamine blends are available in powder and capsule forms; they can improve joint and ligament health and can speed up the recovery process in athletes after injury.

A study conducted by the University of California, School of Medicine in Los Angeles, found that patients who took 2,250 milligrams of MSM daily for six weeks reported an 80 percent reduction in arthritis symptoms.

A study conducted in Texas [24] studied the effects of MSM, glucosamine, and chondroitin in subjects who underwent an exercise and weight-loss program. The participants were administered 1,500 mg of glucosamine, 1,200 mg of chondroitin, and 900 mg of MSM; the combination helped in faster healing and recovery in the participants.

B. Proteolytic enzymes (for use during injury):

These enzymes help in the digestion of proteins. Our body naturally produces protein-digesting enzymes such as trypsin, chymotrypsin, papain, and bromelain; however, proteolytic enzymes not only help in the better digestion of food, but also they help in the reduction of swelling and inflammation.

Many studies provide preliminary evidence that proteolytic enzymes could help in the treatment of various forms of chronic pain, including neck pain and osteoarthritis.

A study of forty-four individuals with sports-related ankle injuries revealed [25] that supplementation of proteolytic enzymes and bioflavonoids resulted in quicker recover from injury; it reduced the period of absence from training by nearly 50 percent.

Recommended proteolytic enzymes:

Bromelain extracted from pineapple stems and papain made from papayas can be purchased as syrups or capsules from health-food stores. Trypsin and chymotrypsin can be used as supplements; they are extracted from the pancreases of various animals.

Gum inflammation: Gingivitis:

Gingivitis is characterized by a persistent and recurrent inflammation and infection of the gums. It presents with swelling and redness of the gum tissue.

Athletes who use mouth breathing during practice or racing are more susceptible to gingivitis.

Many studies have shown that there is a definite connection between gum disease and cardiovascular disease; this happens because the blood vessels in the gums can get infected and carry the bacteria/viruses directly to the heart, thus causing cardiovascular disease.

For this reason it is important to have a regular dental checkup and obtain regular treatment in case of chronic gingivitis.

Power/Super foods:

Aloe vera contains nearly seventy-five potentially active constituents, which include vitamins, enzymes, minerals, sugars, lignin, saponins, salicylic acids, and amino acids. [56–58]

It contains vitamins A (beta-carotene), C, and E, which are antioxidants. It also contains vitamin B12, folic acid, and choline. As an antioxidant, it neutralizes free radicals.

Anti-inflammatory action: Aloe vera has anti-inflammatory properties; studies have shown that aloe vera inhibits the cyclooxygenase pathway and reduces prostaglandin E2 production from arachidonic acid. Recently, the novel anti-inflammatory compound called C-glucosyl chromone was isolated from aloe vera gel extracts.[59]

Effects on the immune system: alprogen present in aloe vera inhibits calcium influx into mast cells, thereby inhibiting the antigen-antibody-mediated release of histamine and leukotriene from mast cells. [60] It lowers free-radical damage by inhibiting the release of reactive oxygen-free radicals from activated human neutrophils.[61]

Antiviral and antitumor activity: these actions are due to stimulation of the immune system and anthraquinones. The anthraquinone aloin inactivates various enveloped viruses such as herpes simplex, varicella zoster, and influenza.[62]

- **Acai** (pronounced "ah-sigh-ee")

  Acai contains anthocyanins and flavonoids.

  Anthocyanins and flavonoids have a powerful antioxidant property, and they help in fighting off the cellular wear and tear created by stress and exertion.

  They counteract the negative effects of free radicals and play a useful role in preventing cancer and heart disease. [54, 55]

  Why is acai considered a power food?

  Acai fruit pulp has a higher antioxidant content than blueberry, blackberry, strawberry, raspberry, or cranberry, with a protein profile similar to an egg, an essential fatty acid profile similar to olive oil, low sugar and low GI, and an ORAC (antioxidant value) higher than blueberries, pomegranate, red wine, and even goji.

  Acai is very popular right now. Acai is available in powdered and packed form.

- **Cherries** (*Prunus avium*)

  Cherries get their rich, deep red color from powerfully antioxidant anthocyanins; they contain free-radical busting ellagic acid (also found in pomegranates) and the flavonoid quercetin.

Cherries are rich in antioxidant content, with no saturated fat, no cholesterol, and low sodium.

A recent research study [26] conducted to evaluate the benefits of cherries for athletes revealed that consumption of 12 oz of cherry juice twice daily helped in the reduction of pain and strength loss after excessive exercise due to its antioxidant effects. [26]

- **Chia seeds (*Salvia hispanica*):**

  Chia seeds are the highest known plant source of omega 3, with eight times more omega 3 than salmon! Unlike other sources of important essential fatty acids (EFA) such as flaxseed or fish oil, chia seeds provide a highly stable form of EFAs due to their powerful naturally occurring antioxidants.

  The antioxidants help in removing free radicals from the body and in fighting inflammation. Chia seeds can be consumed in various forms; making a snack out of chia seeds can keep you healthy and prevent binge eating.

How to incorporate chia seeds into your daily routine:

Super food cereal for athletes:

One of the best ways to incorporate chia seeds into your daily routine is by preparing a chia snack along with other power foods and storing it in a container for long-term use as a snack instead of chips or oily foods.

Here's the recipe for the snack:

Dry ingredients

- 4 cups rolled oats

- 1/2 cup flax meal

- 1/2 cup chia seeds

- 1 cup roasted cashews or almonds or pista

- 3/4 cup dried cherries

- 1 tsp cinnamon

Wet ingredients

- ½ cup black cherry juice concentrate (or regular cherry juice)

- ½ cup canola oil

- ¼ cup blackstrap molasses

- ¼ cup agave syrup

Instructions for preparing the snack:

Warm the oven up to 250 degrees. Combine the wet ingredients and heat them in a microwave for up to two minutes, so that the ingredients are hot. Combine the wet and the dry ingredients; make sure there are no clusters after the ingredients are mixed.

Now bake the ingredients in the oven for around thirty-five to forty-five minutes. Remove the ingredients and let them cool. Store the snack in a bottle or Tupperware container.

Goji berries (Chinese wolfberry or gou qi zi): Goji berries are healthy snack foods that taste like cherry.

Benefits of goji berries:

Goji contains

- twenty-one minerals,

- super-high concentrations of vitamin C,

- vitamin A,

- complete protein (eighteen amino acids), and

- an ORAC (antioxidant) score of 25,300! (For comparison, blueberries score 2,400; green tea, 1,686; and broccoli, 890.)

Coconuts:

Young coconuts are one of the highest sources of electrolytes in nature. Electrolytes are ionized salts in our cells that transport energy through-out the body; they also help in better nerve conduction and ion exchange for good muscle function.

Blueberries:

Blueberries are often considered a super food (or super fruit) because they contain significant amounts of antioxidants, anthocyanins, vitamin C, manganese, and dietary fiber.

Green tea

Green tea is one of the most studied natural supplements; for more than a decade, researchers have been studying the effects of green tea and its role in fighting off cancer, diabetes, heart disease, and its burning fat by lowering levels of cholesterol.

Green tea contains powerful antioxidants known as catechins, which help in scavenging free radicals from the body, thereby protecting the DNA from being exposed to harmful chemicals that can lead to tumor and clot formation.

Green tea also acts as a dilator and makes blood vessels less vulnerable for clogging. Green tea is considered to have more health benefits than black tea due to its minimal processing; the tea leaves are withered and steamed instead of being fermented. This process of preparation helps the tea preserve its catechins.

White tea:

Like black and green tea, white tea comes from Chinese *Camellia sinensis* plant; however, white tea is derived from the delicate buds and younger leaves of the plant.

These buds and leaves are allowed to wither in natural sunlight before they are lightly processed to prevent oxidation or further tea processing. This preserves the characteristic flavor of the white tea.

White tea also contains a higher ratio of catechins, which help cardio-vascular function. White tea also has antibacterial and antiviral properties. Studies conducted at Pace University [27] showed that white tea helps in slowing down the speed of bacterial and viral growth, thereby reducing the incidence of staphylococcus and streptococcus infections, pneumonia, fungus growth, and even dental plaque.

Studies conducted at the Kingstone University [28, 29] revealed that white tea has anti-inflammatory and anti-collagenase properties, which help in fighting rheumatoid arthritis, inflammatory conditions, and aging.

Recommended stores:

HerbaSway: http://www.herbasway.com/

HerbaSway's commitment is to support a well-balanced diet and exercise plan with all natural supplements that can be enjoyed daily and easily.

The company wanted to go beyond the typical multivitamin pill and really focus on specific nutritional goals. After a great deal of research, they decided to develop liquid concentrates, so that they were better absorbed into the bloodstream as well as easier and more enjoyable to take every day. The store has several traditional herbal combinations in a liquid forms, so they can be consumed and absorbed easily.

iherb: http://www.iherb.com/

iHerb sells nutritional supplements and other healthy products both domestically and internationally. iHerb carries one of the largest selections of high-quality nutritional products in the world and provides all top brands and natural herbal products at a cheap price; its shipping policy is unrivaled, and it delivers products at your doorstep in record time (usually within forty-eight to seventy-two hours in the US; coupon code: NCM302—$10 off)

Dark chocolate:

These benefits are from flavonoids, which act as antioxidants. Antioxidants protect the body from aging caused by free radicals, which can cause damage and lead to heart disease. Dark chocolate contains a large number of antioxidants (nearly eight times the number found in strawberries). Flavonoids also help relax blood pressure through the production of nitric oxide and balance certain hormones in the body.

Many different vitamins and minerals that can enhance your health are found in dark chocolate. Dark chocolate is known to have high concentrations of magnesium, iron, copper, and potassium.

Copper and potassium play an important role in preventing heart disease and brain stroke. The magnesium found in dark chocolate helps lower blood pressure and the risks of Type II diabetes.

Dark chocolate also has theobromine, the substance that acts as a mild stimulant, suppresses coughs, and helps harden the tooth enamel, so, unlike other forms of milk chocolate, the theobromine in dark chocolate helps reduce the risk of tooth cavities.

Chocolate contains phenylethylamine (PEA); this chemical is released whenever a person falls in love; therefore, eating chocolate helps improve the mood by releasing endorphins and PEA.

Recommended for Athletes

1) Douglas Labs: Klean Athlete series http://kleanathlete.com/

2) Herbalife: 24 Series for protein/hydration/recovery

http://catalog.herbalife.com/Catalog/en-US/Energy-Fitness/ Herbalife24

3) Optimum Nutrition: For Whey and Casein protein

http://www.optimumnutrition.com/products/100-whey-gold-standard-p-201.html?zenid=7e85c657ad0176b60c06c59c3187dd18

References:

(1)   Ping-Delfos, W., Soares, M. Diet Induced Thermogenesis, Fat Oxidation and Food Intake Following Sequential Meals: Influence of Calcium and Vitamin D. *Clinical Nutrition*. 30, 376–383, 2011.

(2)   Weaver, K. L, Ivester, P; Chilton, J. A.; Wilson, M. D.; Pandey, P.; Chilton, F. H. The content of favorable and unfavorable polyunsaturated fatty acids found in commonly eaten fish *J Am Diet Assoc*.108:1178–1185, 2008.

(3)   *Am J Clin Nutr.* 2004.

(4)   Ostund, R. E. Phytosterols, cholesterol absorption and healthy diets. *Lipids.* e-pub 9 January 2007.

(5)   http://www.nhs.uk/Conditions/vitamins-minerals/Pages/vita-mins-minerals.aspx

(6)   Nieman, D.C.; Henson, D. A.; Davis, J. M., et al. Quercetin's influence on exercise-induced changes in plasma cytokines and muscle and leukocyte cytokine mRNA. *J Appl Physiol* 103:1728–35, 2007.

(7)   Nieman, D. C.; Henson, D. A.; Gross, S. J.; et al. Quercetin reduces illness but not immune perturbations after intensive exercise. *Med Sci Sports Exerc* 39:1561–9, 2007.

(8)   Linus Pauling Institute: Resveratrol.

(9)   http://www.webmd.com/heart-disease/resveratrol-supplements

(10)   Antioxidant lozenge could help ward off flu. www.reutershealth.com (accessed 19 April 2000).

(11)   Powers, S. K.; Ji, L. L.; Leeuwenburgh, C. Exercise training-induced alterations in skeletal muscle antioxidant capacity: A brief review. *Med Sci Sports Exerc* 31:987–97,1999.

(12)   Hiller, W. D., et al. Medical and physiological considerations in triathlons. *Am J Sports Med* Mar(2):164–7,1987.

(13)   Cordova, A. Behaviour of zinc in physical exercise: A special reference to immunity and fatigue. *Neurosci Biobehav Rev* Fall 19(3):439–45,1995.

(14)   Cordova, A., et al. Effect of training on zinc metabolism: changes in serum and sweat zinc concentrations in sportsmen. *Ann Nutr Metab* 42(5):274–821998;.

(15)   Barrie, S. A., et al. Comparative absorption of zinc picolinate, zinc citrate and zinc gluconate in humans. *Agents Actions* 21(1-2):223–8,1987.

(16)   Rohde, T., et al. Effect of glutamine supplementation on changes in the immune system induced by repeated exercise. *Med Sci Sports Exerc* 30(6):856–62, 1998.

(17)   Newsholme, E. A., et al. The proposed role of glutamine in some cells of the immune system and speculative consequences for the whole animal. *Nutrition.* Jul–Aug; 13(7–8):728–30, 1997.

(18)   Rohde, T., et al. Effect of glutamine supplementation on changes in the immune system induced by repeated exercise. *Med Sci Sports Exerc* 30(6):856–62, 1998.

(19)   Castell, L. M., et al. Does glutamine have a role in reducing infections in athletes? *Eur J Appl Physiol* 73(5):488–90, 1996.

(20)   Cox, A. J.; Pyne, D. B.; Saunders, P. U.; and Fricker, P. A. Oral administration of the probiotic lactobacillus fermentum VR1-003 and mucosal immunity in endurance athletes. *British Journal of Sports Medicine* (2007) http://news.bbc.co.uk/2/hi/health/7243006.stm

(21)   *Journal of the International Society of Sports Nutrition*; December 2008,   Electronic   Pre-publication.http://www.nutritionexpress.com/article+index/vitamins+supplements+a-z/showarticle.aspx?id=1137

(22)   Nichols, A. W. Probiotics and athletic performance: A systematic review. *Curr Sports Med Rep.*6(4):269–73, 2007.

(23) Berg, A.; et al. J. Influence of echinacin (EC31) treatment on the exercise-induced immune response in athletes. *Journal of Clinical Research* 1: 367–380, 1998.

(24) Magrans, T., et al. Effects of diet type and supplementation of glucosamine, chondroitin, and MSM on body composition, functional status, and markers of health in women with knee osteoarthritis initiating a resistance-based exercise and weight loss program. *Journal of the International Society of Sports Nutrition.* 8(8), 2011.

(25) http://hcasaludinternacional.com/your-health/?/21432/Sports-Injuries#P3

(26) Connolly, D.A., et al. Efficacy of a tart cherry juice blend in preventing the symptoms of muscle damage. *Br J Sports Med* 40:679–83; discussion 683, 2006.

(27) Pace University. New study shows that white tea has an inhibitory effect on various pathogenic bacteria, fungi and bacterial virus. Retrieved 23 July 2012.

(28) *Science Daily.* White tea could keep you healthy and looking young. Retrieved 12 June 2011.

(29) Thring; Tamsyn, S. A.; Hili, P.; Naughton, D. P. Anti-collagenase, anti-elastase and anti-oxidant activities of extracts from 21 plants. *BMC Complementary and Alternative Medicine* 9. doi:10.1186/1472-6882-9-27. (2009).

(29b) Brotherhood 1984.

(30) http://www.ausport.gov.au/ais/nutrition/factsheets/hydration/how_much_do_athletes_sweat

(31) http://www.fifa.com/mm/document/afdeveloping/medi-cal/4.6.%20hydration%20p%2020-21_1493.pdf

(32) Kerksick et al., 2008, p. 4.

(33) The Sports, Cardiovascular, and Wellness Nutrition (SCAN) dietetic practice group of the American Academy of Nutrition and Dietetics.

(34) Kerksick et al., 2008, p. 9.

(35) Kerksick et al., 2008, p. 7.

(36) Jurimae, J.; Jurimae, T.; and Purge, P. Plasma testosterone and cortisol responses to prolonged sculling in male competitive rowers. *Journal of Sports Sciences* 19, 893–898, 2001.

Duke, J. W.; Rubin, D. A.; Daly, W.; and Hackney, A.C. Influence of prolonged exercise on the 24-hour free testosterone-cortisol ratio hormonal profile. *Medicina Sportiva* 11(2): 48–50, 2007.

(37) Fry, R. W.; Morton, A. R.; Keast, D. Overtraining in athletes: an update. *Sports Medicine* 12 (1): 32–65, 1991.

(38) Curr Atheroscler Rep. 2004 Nov;6(6):461-7.Omega-3 fatty acids and inflammation. Mori TA, Beilin LJ. School of Medicine and Pharmacology—Royal Perth Hospital Unit, The University of Western Australia, Medical Research Foundation Building, Perth, Western Australia 6847, Australia. tmori@cyllene.uwa.edu.au

(39) Natural Medicines Comprehensive Database website: "Elderberry." Natural Standard Patient Monograph: "Elderberry."

(40) Lindeman 1990.

(41)   De Wijn and Van Erp-Baart 1980; Khoo et al. 1987; Van Erp-Baart et al. 1989; Lindeman, 1990; Burke et al. 1991; Hawley and Williams 1991; Butterworth et al. 1994). Burke et al. 1991.

(42)   Hawley and Williams 1991.

(43)   Hawley, J. A.; Burk, L. M. Effect of meal frequency and timing on physical performance. *British Journal of Nutrition* 77, Suppl. 1, 591–5103 44, 1997.

(45)   Sherman et al. 1989.

(46)   Noakes, T. D. Fluid replacement during exercise. *Exerc. Sports Sci. Rev.* 21:297–330.3. 1993.

Mathews, D. K.; Fox, E. L.; and Tanzi, D. Physiological responses during exercise and recovery. 1969.

(47)   http://www.afpafitness.com/articles/articles-and-newletters/research-articles-index/athletes-sports-conditioning/why-water-is-the-most-important-nutrient-for-endurance-athletes/

(48)   Jeukendrup 2004, 2008; Jeukendrup et al. 1997.

(49)   Coyle et al. 1986.

(50)   Keizer et al. 1987a.

(51)   Burke, L.M.; Cox, G. R.; Culmmings, N. K.; and Desbrow, B. Guidelines for daily carbohydrate intake: Do athletes achieve them?

(52)   Carroll, C. Protein and exercise, In Rosenbloom, C., ed. *Sports Nutrition: A Guide for the Professional Working with Active People.* 3rd ed. Chicago: The American Dietetic Association; 2000.

(53) Lemon, P. Is increased dietary protein necessary or beneficial for individuals with a physically active lifestyle? *Nutrition Reviews* 54:S169–S175,1996.

(54) Natural Medicines: Comprehensive Database: Acai Monograph.

(55) http://www.webmd.com/diet/acai-berries-and-acai-berry-juice-what-are-the-health-benefits

(56) Atherton, P. Aloe vera revisited. *Br J Phytother*. 4:76–83, 1998.

(57) Shelton M. Aloe vera, its chemical and therapeutic properties. *Int J Dermatol*. 30:679–83, 1991.

(58) Atherton P. *The essential aloe vera: The actions and the evidence.* 2nd ed. 1997.

(59) Hutter, J. A., et al. Anti-inflammatory C-glucosyl chromone from Aloe barbadensis. *J Nat Prod*. 59:541–3, 1996.

(60) Ro, J. Y., et al. Inhibitory mechanism of aloe single component (Alprogen) on mediator release in guinea pig lung mast cells activated with specific antigen-antibody reactions. *J Pharmacol Exp Ther.* 292:114–21, 2000.

(61) Hart, L. A., et al. Effects of low molecular constituents from aloe vera gel on oxidative metabolism and cytotoxic and bactericidal activities of human neutrophils. *Int J Immunopharmacol.* 12:427–34, 1990.

(62) Sydiskis, R. J., et al. Inactivation of enveloped viruses by anthraquinones extracted from plants. *Antimicrob Agents Chemother*. 35:2463–6, 1991.

Recommended reading:

Beals, K.; Manore, M. Nutritional status of female athletes with sub-clinical eating disorders. *J Am Diet Assoc.*;98:419–425,1998.

Chandler, R, Byrne H, Patterson J, Ivy J. Dietary supplements affect the anabolic hormones after weight training exercise. *J Appl Physiol.*76:839–845,1994.

Clin Sports Med. R007 Jan;26(1):17–36.

Kleiner, S. Bodybuilding. In Rosenbloom, C., ed. *Sports Nutrition: A Guide for the Professional Working with Active People.* 3rd ed. Chicago: The American Dietetic Association; 2000.

Tipton, K. D.; Witard, O. C. Protein requirements and recommendations for athletes: Relevance of ivory-tower arguments for practical recommendations.

The Fifth Pillar

Physical

The Fifth Pillar: Physical

ADDING CHIROPRACTIC, MASSAGE, YOGA, AND PHYSICAL THERAPY CAN make a huge difference with injury prevention and recovery. Moreover, maintaining proper biomechanics, muscle symmetry, and balance are essential.

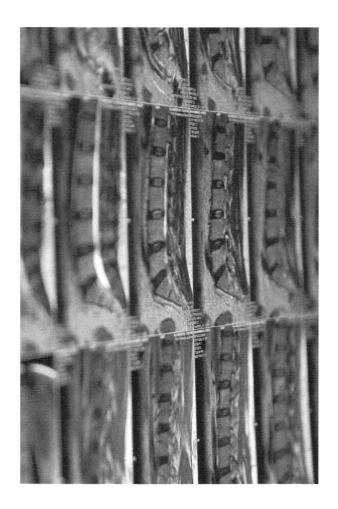

The chiropractic elements can include the following:

- spinal manipulation

- extra spinal manipulation

- soft-tissue techniques—ART, Graston, myofacial release, SASTM

- taping: McConnel, Kinesio tape, SpiderTech, ROCKTAPE, specific proprioceptive response technique (SPRT), Tim Brown

- fascial manipulation

Spinal Manipulation [1]:

Spinal manipulation, performed mostly by chiropractors, has been used for a long time. Athletes have sought out the chiropractic profession for help with injuries and improved performance based on its reputation as an excellent drug-free holistic approach to care. In fact, today most professional teams have at least one chiropractor on staff, and the USA Olympic team takes several chiropractors to each of the games. In fact, Dr. Moreau, a chiropractor, is the director of Sports Medicine Clinics for the United States Olympic Committee, in which he leads the multiple-disciplinary sports-medicine teams at all three Olympic training centers. Spinal manipulation or manual therapy is quickly becoming the preferred method of treatment for athletes who experience spinal problems. Spinal manipulation works on the premise of restoring motion and increasing flexibility of ligamentous adhesions, muscle spasm, disk nutrition, and central nervous system endorphin systems.

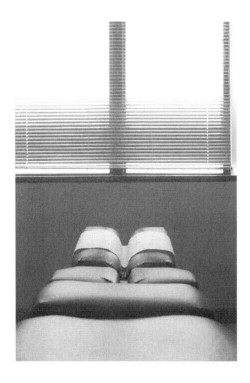

Spinal manipulation uses quick and safe maneuvers to facilitate movements in joints that exhibit a decreased range of movement; this reduces the pain associated with the joint and can be used to increase motion in joints with a limited range of movement.

The concept of joint barriers has been developed to differentiate among exercise therapy, mobilization, and manipulation. Research trials [1] reveal that spinal manipulation is beneficial in relieving or reducing the duration of acute low-back pain and acute neck pain but has much less effect on chronic low-back pain and neck pain.

Evidence suggests that manipulation increases certain parameters of motion of the spine, but this evidence is not yet conclusive. There are a wide variety of manipulative procedures that are utilized to manipulate the spine to increase range of motion, and the selection of the procedures is based on manual diagnostic skills. Research studies [2] have demonstrated a trend toward lower-limb injury prevention with a significant reduction in primary lower-limb muscle strains and weeks missed due to non-contact knee injuries through the addition of a sports chiropractic intervention to the current best-practice management.

It's been found [3] that the underlying mechanisms explaining the benefits of SMT appear to be multi-factorial. Both spinal stiffness characteristics and LM recruitment changes appear to play a role.

Commonly used techniques for spinal manipulation include flexion distraction technique; in this technique a flexion distraction table is used to manipulate the lumbar and thoracic spine. The flexion table can move in all directions (up, down, side to side) and provide traction; this helps in mobilizing the spinal joints and reducing the spasm in soft tissues. Many research studies have shown that lumbar traction techniques help in reducing intra-discal pressure, improving the hydration of degenerated discs and decreasing the security of disk herniations.

Extra spinal manipulation:

Extra spinal manipulation is defined as the application of manipulation or mobilization to joints other than those of the spine; i.e., shoulder, elbow, wrist/hand/finger, hip, knee, and ankle/foot/toe.

It is generally recommended for patients with neuro-musculoskeletal disorders involving the shoulder, elbow, wrist/hand, hip, knee, ankle, and foot.

Several factors are involved in the recovery process of an athlete suffering from joint pains; one of the most crucial elements to recovery is joint play. Joint play is described as that degree of end movement (paraphysiologic) beyond active and passive motion that cannot be attained through regular voluntary movement.

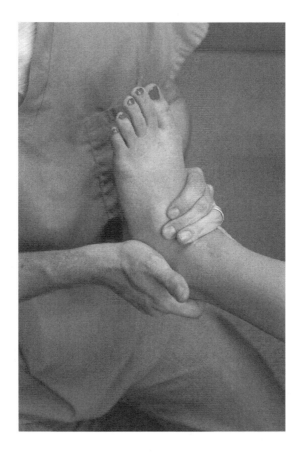

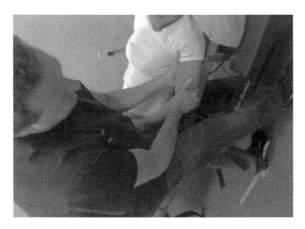

Normal joint play usually does not require any manipulation; however, hypo-mobility requires the use of specific manipulation techniques to reduce the restriction of movement.

Soft-tissue techniques:

<u>Active release technique (ART):</u>
History:

ART has been developed, refined, and patented by P. Michael Leahy, DC, CCSP. Dr. Leahy noticed that his patients' symptoms seemed to be related to changes in their soft tissue that could be felt by hand. By observing how muscles, fascia, tendons, ligaments, and nerves responded to different types of work, Dr. Leahy was able to consistently resolve over 90 percent of his patients' problems. He now teaches and certifies health care providers all over the world to use ART.

Premise: the basic technique is to shorten the tissue, apply a contact tension and lengthen the tissue or make it slide relative to the adjacent tissue.

Many different musculoskeletal conditions can benefit from ART. Most of these conditions result from overuse of muscles, which then leads to

- overused muscles (and other soft tissues),

- acute conditions (pulls, tears, collisions, etc.), and

- accumulation of small tears (micro-trauma) and not getting enough oxygen (hypoxia).

These can eventually lead to muscle spasm, scar-tissue formation, and subsequent reduction of function.

Below is the cumulative injury cycle formulated by Dr. Leahy to describe the escalating patterns of pain, injury, and formation of adhesions that occur with many repetitive-strain injuries.

Every ART session is actually a combination of examination and treatment. The ART provider uses his or her hands to evaluate the texture, tightness, and movement of muscles, fascia, tendons, ligaments, and nerves. Abnormal tissues are treated by combining precisely directed tension with very specific patient movements.

The active release technique works according to the law of repetitive motion.

Active release technique can be used for two main purposes:

- Injury care: To resolve soft tissue problems caused by repetitive strain injuries, tissue hypoxia, joint dysfunctions, etc. It helps in treating the specific area of injury as well as related structures.

- Performance care: To correct areas of restricted action, and for biomechanical analysis of gait and motion.

IASTM (instrument-assisted soft-tissue mobilization techniques)

The Graston Technique:

The Graston technique (GT) is a therapeutic method used for the diagnosis and treatment of disorders related to the skeletal muscles and connective tissue. The therapist uses six stainless-steel tools of different shapes and sizes to palpate the patient's body and to resolve the adhesions detected in the muscles and tendons.

The therapist will use different variables to achieve different treatment outcomes; these variables include changes in stroke direction, stroke amplitude, stroke rate, amount of surface contact, amount of applied pressure; depth of penetration, angle of application, treatment frequency, and treatment duration. It is hypothesized that Graston restarts the inflammatory process and stimulates the healing cascade through the introduction of micro-trauma.

There may be associated bruising noticed after treatment; this is temporary and is produced by localized micro-trauma and associated scar-tissue breakdown.

Graston can be integrated with other techniques and modalities. It's critical to follow the treatment with stretching and strengthening; the treatment may also end with cryotherapy.

The technique can be used after obtaining a license from the Graston Technique Institute. It's important to note that this license is available only for health-care professionals.

(More information about training is available at www.grastontechnique.com)

The training is delivered through two modules: M1 and M2

Module 1 involves Graston Technique® basic training.

Module 2 involves upper and lower quadrant techniques.

Research studies [5,6] conducted on GT have shown that the controlled micro-trauma induced through GT protocol increases the amount of fibroblasts produced at the treated area. That amount of inflammation to the scar tissue helps initiate the healing cascade. The structure of the tissue is rearranged, and damaged tissue is replaced by new tissue. Ice is then applied to reduce the pain, and exercise is implemented to increase function and range of motion.

Other clinical studies continue to document the success of GT, generally achieving better outcomes when compared to traditional therapies, and resolving injuries that have failed to respond to other therapies.

Benefits of Graston Technique:

The technique is aimed at separating and breaking down collagen cross-links; it also splays and stretches connective tissue and muscle fibers.

Other significant benefits of Graston Technique:

- increases skin temperature

- facilitates reflex changes in the chronic muscle holding pattern

- alters spinal reflux activity (facilitated segment)

- increases the rate and amount of blood flow to and from the area

- increases cellular activity in the region, including fibro-blasts and mast cells

- increases histamine response secondary to mast cell activity

- decreases overall time of treatment

- fosters faster rehabilitation/recovery

- reduces need for anti-inflammatory medication

- resolves chronic conditions thought to be permanent

Sound-assisted soft tissue mobilization:

Sound-assisted soft tissue mobilization (SASTM) uses a set of special instruments to break down scar tissue and fascial restrictions. It is a type of manual therapy that is effective in reducing pain and restoring function in athletes suffering with spine, neck, and extremity disorders.

This type of treatment originates from the two-thousand-year-old tra-ditional Chinese medicine technique called *Gua Sha,* which means "to scrape toxins."

How it was developed:

David Graston developed SASTM to assist in his own recovery from carpal tunnel and a knee injury he suffered while skiing. Graston worked with a group of medical doctors, therapists, and athletic trainers to perfect the technique and the tools necessary for successful practice.

Graston continues to work with medical doctors, chiropractors, therapists, professional athletes, and trainers to produce improvements in range of motion, flexibility, recovery time, and performance through the use of SASTM; the technique has been upgraded many times.

Benefits:

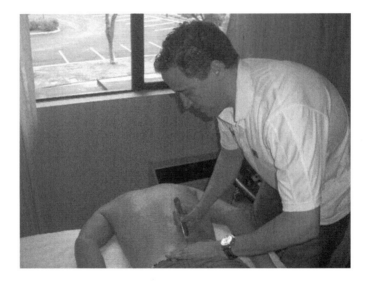

It's been found that adhesions and scar tissue usually develop after surgery, immobilization, or repeated strain. SASTM helps in breaking down the scar tissue and allows your body to return back to healthy function. SASTM is effective for a number of physical concerns:

- relief from tendonitis

- recovery from carpal tunnel syndrome

- recovery from ankle strains/sprains

- oxygenates tissues

- detoxification of stagnant tissue

- increased range of motion and pain relief from hamstring injuries

- relief from hip- and knee-replacement dysfunction and pain

- relief from shin-splint pain

How it works:

The tools used in SASTM are specifically designed to treat soft-tissue disorders that may have developed as a result of surgery, immobilization, repetitive strains, or direct injury. The treatment starts with the application of cream or oil to the body and then scraping the skin with the flat tool to promote blood and lymphatic circulation; it also helps in removing toxic heat and facilitates pain relief. In the SASTM method, the therapist usually works beneath the level of skin to the fibrotic tissue to locate and release adhesions and restrictions in the body with friction and pressure.

The use of the tools in the affected soft tissues causes a local inflammatory response or micro-trauma. This response initiates the reabsorption of fibrotic or excessive scar tissue and facilitates a cascade of immune-system cell flow to the treated area. These cells begin to flush away cellular debris and begin the process of repair and restoration to normal function.

Instruments used in SASTM effectively break down fascial restrictions and scar tissue. The ergonomic design of these instruments provides the clinician with the ability to locate restrictions through sound waves. This allows the clinician to treat the affected area with the appropriate amount of pressure, due to a square-surface concept.

The introduction of controlled microtrauma to affected soft tissue structure causes the stimulation of a local inflammatory response.

Microtrauma initiates reabsorption of inappropriate fibrosis or excessive scar tissue and facilitates a cascade of healing activities resulting in remodeling of affected soft tissue structures. Adhesions within the soft tissue, which may have developed as a result of surgery, immobilization, repeated strain, or other mechanisms, are broken down, allowing full functional restoration to occur.

Based on literature and years of clinical research, here is a list of disorders that instrument-assisted soft tissue mobilization has most effectively been used for in the restoration of function and pain reduction.

ConnecTX™:

One of the newest instrument-assisted soft tissue mobilization tecneques is ConnecTX™ Therapy, which is a trademarked, instrument-assisted, soft-tissue mobilization technique that employs newly established protocols and a prescriptive exercise program to assist manual therapists in the detection and treatment of various connective tissue (CT) disorders. Certified ConnecTX™ instruction is affordably priced and presented by experienced ConnecTX™ clinicians. The ConnecTX™ instrument is uniquely designed to comfortably fit the curves of the body, giving clinicians broad access for examination and treatment. The instrument's ergonomic design incorporates a brushed, nonslip surface that reduces fatigue within the clinician's hands and provides improved kinesthetic feedback for treatment application. ConnecTX™ Therapy emollient is specifically formulated to work with the instrument and provides a smooth, friction-appropriate interface between the patient's skin and the instrument.

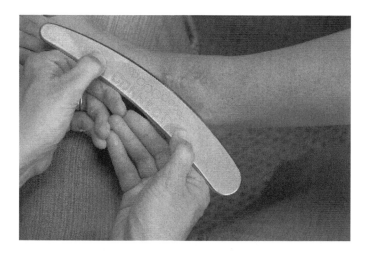

The body of knowledge that supports ConnecTX™ protocols is constantly changing; therefore, a patient-centered-outcome research initiative is already under way, wherein New York Chiropractic College's (NYCC) research department will collect clinical data from ConnecTX™ practitioners and monitor effectiveness and document any adverse reactions. ConnecTX™ certified doctors will play a significant role in the ongoing development of the protocols, maintaining their certification by furnishing case studies and participating in the collection of clinical information. As patient results are examined, new information may be gathered from researchers and practitioners who use the instrument consistent with existing protocols and best practices. The amassed information will be used to create educational materials for downloading and distribution to ConnecTX™ certified practitioners and their patients.

Doctors certified in ConnecTX Therapy will become part of a ConnecTX™ community of scholars who maintain their certification by furnishing case studies and participating in the collection of clinical information. A patient-centered outcome research initiative is under way wherein NYCC's research department collects clinical data from ConnecTX practitioners in order to monitor and document effectiveness and to assist in the ongoing development of ConnecTX protocols. The amassed body of science will be used to create educational materials that may be downloaded and distributed to certified practitioners and their patients.

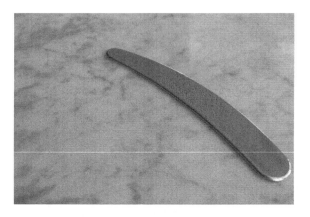

Taping techniques:

There are many types of taping techniques used in the United States; these are some of the more common:

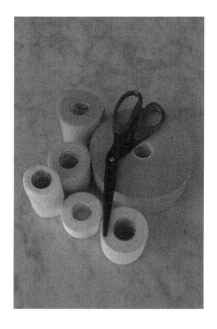

- white athletic taping

- McConnell® taping

- Kinesio Taping® method

- ROCKTAPE method

- SpiderTech method

1. White athletic taping:

This is the most common type of taping technique used in the United States. The tape is very rigid and also requires a pre-tape to be applied for enhanced skin protection. There is a high chance of irritation due to trapped moisture; tight compression of skin, muscles, and joints; and high latex content of the tape. The tape is mainly used during sport; it may be applied prior to the sporting event, worn for a short period of time, and removed at the end of the game. This tape does not have any rehabilitative use.

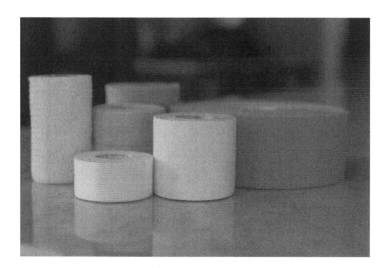

2. McConnell® taping:

This form of taping uses a brace or a strap that consists of a highly rigid, highly adhesive cotton mesh tape (EnduraTape®, LeukoTape®).

This tape is commonly used for treatment of patellofemoral and shoulder subluxation, as well as lumbar, foot, and hip impingement.

It is left on the skin for a shorter period of time (less than eighteen hours), because it has a very strong suffocating and constricting effect; it may also cause adverse skin reactions. The method is usually used for neuromuscular reeducation of the affected tissues and joints.

Jenny McConnell, PT, GDMT, founder of the McConnell Institute, developed the method bearing her name for the treatment of patellofemoral pain syndrome. It involves assessing the orientation of the patella, determining which components need to be corrected, taping the patella into alignment, and specifically retraining the appropriate muscles.

She has since developed methods for the treatment of the shoulder. Her method can be summarized as a bracing technique that is primarily used for neuromuscular reeducation. The tape required is again a two-part combination consisting of a latex-free elastic underwrap (white) and highly rigid/adhesive tape (brown). Two highly accepted options are LeukoTape P® with Cover-Roll® stretch, or EnduraSPORTS Tape with EnduraFIX tape.

3. Kinesio® taping method:

Kinesio taping uses a water-resistant, elastic, latex-free tape for achieving the therapeutic and rehabilitative purposes.

Kinesio taping is regarded as a definitive and rehabilitative taping technique that enhances the body's natural healing process by providing support and stability to muscles and joints; it allows for a good range of motion and provides soft tissue manipulation for extended periods, thus prolonging the benefits associated with this form of therapy.

The therapist uses a specific tape known as Kinesio Tex Gold for this purpose; the tape is elastic, resilient (stays up to three to five days), waterproof, and suitable for all ages. It takes minimal time to apply the tape, and it can be removed very easily.

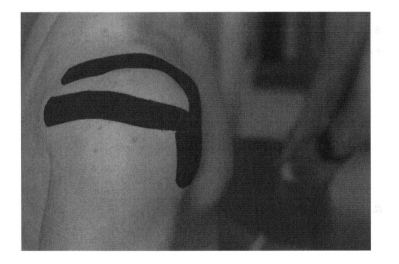

Kinesio taping has several benefits: it helps in reducing pain, enhancing performance, retraining the neuromuscular system, reducing chances of injury, and promoting lymphatic flow. It is used to treat a variety of orthopedic, neuromuscular, neurological, and other medical conditions. It has the dual benefit of both providing physical support and rehabilitation. The Kinesio tapes are latex-free; therefore, they can be worn for days at a time.

The regular athletic tape is usually rigid and is designed to act as a stabilizing force with an intention of supporting the associated joints; it also limits the mobility and range of movement of the affected joint.

The unique features of the Kinesio Tex® tape allow it to stretch when applied. This lifting affect forms convolutions in the skin, thus increasing interstitial space and allowing for a decrease in inflammation of the affected areas; this in turn produces a decrease in pressure within the dermis, the layer of tissue underneath the skin.

This effect is very helpful, because the dermis contains many blood vessels, lymph vessels, and neural receptors that are responsible for sensing pain and movement. The reduced pressure increases the cellular interstitial space, which allows for increased blood flow and lymphatic drainage. By targeting different receptors within the somatosensory system, Kinesio® Tex Tape alleviates pain.

The nervous system in the dermis is also affected by the Kinesio tape, because it creates a gentle sensory stimulation for all sensory receptors. The tape can therefore have the effect of blocking the sensation of pain (nociception) as well as stimulating fine-motor control of musculature (mechanoreceptors). In essence this means decreased pressure leading to decreased pain and an improvement in muscle function.

The method:

The Kinesio taping method consists of taping over and around muscles in order to assist and give support to muscles or to prevent over-contraction of muscles, depending on patient presentation. Kinesio taping can easily be integrated into a patients' existing treatment plan.

The Kinesio taping method can also be combined with Active Release® technique and Graston technique.

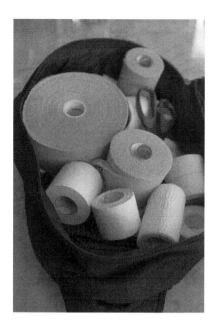

History of Kinesio taping:

Kinesio taping was invented by Dr. Kenso Kase, a Japanese chiropractor, nearly thirty years ago. The tape has undergone several modifications, and it's different from other forms of athletic taping. The Kinesio tape can stretch up to 140 percent, and therefore it allows for a free range of motion after the tape is applied.

This tape facilitates easy movements in the joints and enables the athletes to engage in their typical daily activities or athletic pursuits without hindrance.

In fact, the Kinesio taping technique is employed by hundreds of athletes in many countries on both the amateur and professional levels. Many athletes around the world used the tape during the Beijing Olympics.

The Kinesio® Tex Tape is specifically applied to the patient after an evaluation of his/her specific needs. The findings of the clinical evaluation or assessment will help the therapist choose the specific type of the Kinesio® Tex Tape application and other adjunctive treatments and modalities.

With the utilization of single *I* strips or modifications in the shape of an *X*, *Y*, or other specialized shapes, as well as the direction and amount of stretch placed on the tape at time of application, Kinesio® Tex Tape can be applied in hundreds of ways and has the ability to reeducate the neuromuscular system, reduce pain and inflammation, enhance performance, prevent injury, promote good circulation and healing, and assist in returning.

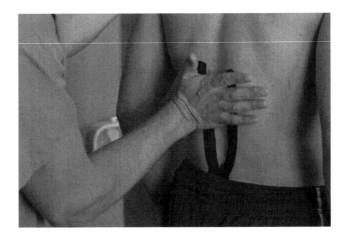

The Kinesio tape is very versatile; the desired effect of treatment can be altered by changing how, where, and with what tension the tape is applied.

Many different types of correctional Kinesio taping techniques can be practiced, depending upon the specific condition that needs to be treated.

The correctional techniques are chosen to achieve specific mechanical, lymphatic, ligament/tendon, fascial, space, and functional outcomes.

These numerous applications and varieties available with the Kinesio tape enhance the ability of the tape to address musculoskeletal issues.

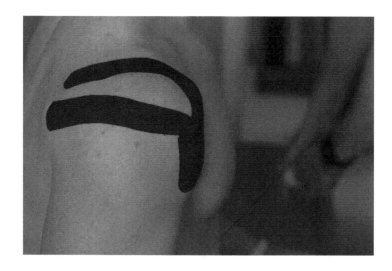

Tips for achieving the best results with Kinesio taping:

a. Ensure that the skin is free of oil, sweat, or lotion prior to application.

b. Ensure the tape is placed in the right position and then activate the heat-sensitive glue by rubbing up and down the surface of the tape.

c. Avoid extreme stretching of the tape during application to avoid skin irritation.

d. Apply approximately one hour prior to activity or shower to allow the glue to adhere properly.

e. Skin irritation is extremely rare, but care should be taken with hyper-sensitive skin patients.

ROCKTAPE:

ROCKTAPE is a brand name for a series of tapes that are specially designed to enhance performance and recovery and are engineered to meet the demands of endurance athletes such as runners, swimmers, and cyclists.

Unlike regular compression garments and tapes, ROCKTAPE can be used both to apply compression to promote recovery, or to apply decompression to relieve pain and swelling. ROCKTAPE is used in many countries and is preferred for treating common injuries such as shin splints, lower back and knee issues (ACL/MCL/meniscus), shoulder impingement, broken collarbones, and tennis elbow.

ROCKTAPE also offers a POWER Taping method that can be used by athletes to enhance performance by mitigating fatigue and promoting better form. It is used to treat lower back issues and swelling associated with pregnancy. It uses the best 6/12 nylon, cotton, and acrylic adhesives, which are latex-free and are FDA/CE-approved.

The tape works on the mechanism of core stabilization and proprioception. Core stabilization leads to better diaphragm use, and proprioception leads to better form.

The tape has a 190 percent elasticity, which allows the athlete to enjoy a fuller and better range of motion.

Benefits of ROCKTAPE:

1) Increased awareness of the sensorimotor (proprioceptive) system—the power-taping manual suggests that the tape helps the brain become more aware of its body position and trains the receptors to adjust the body's position naturally; the tactile nature of the tape increases awareness of the body's own location and movements.

2) Inflammation control—the tape helps lift the skin away from the underlying fascia, which holds blood and lymph vessels and nerves. This extra space relieves fluid congestion, reduces inflammation and pain, and allows for increased blood flow and therefore accelerates healing. Due to

reduced inflammation, the pain receptors are not activated; this allows the athlete to perform at high levels without experiencing much pain.

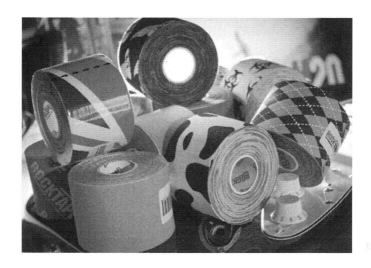

3) Works the kinetic chain—PowerTaping works on the concept of muscles acting as parts in a chain. Thomas W. Myers calls this phenomenon the "all one fascia" in his book *Anatomy Trains*. It signifies that you are always taping the movement pattern in the body and not the isolated body parts.

4) Snap-back mechanism—The tape has a "snap back" mechanism: the elastic recoil of the ROCKTAPE assists in bringing muscles back to their original position efficiently when a movement is being completed. This results in improved performance.

Highlights of ROCKTAPE functions

- rehabilitation

- edema control

- postural control

- improved sports performance

More information and instructional videos are available at the website www.rocktape.com.

SpiderTech Kinesiology Tape (available at http://www.spidertech.com):

SpiderTech tape is a nonmedicated cotton kinesiology tape that you apply to your body wherever it hurts. SpiderTech provides convenient, standardized, and easy-to-use precut kinesiology tape applications called Spiders.

How does it work?

The tape, made with hypoallergenic acrylic glue, is manufactured to be the same weight, thickness, and elasticity as the skin and is therefore able to integrate with the body's sensory system naturally.

There are three possible categories of effect which have been identified, depending on the method of application and the therapeutic outcome desired:

1. Structurally:
- The elastic property of the tape dynamically supports better postural positions.
- Prevent harmful ranges of motion without a hard-end feel.
- Reduce strain on affected muscle.

2. Neurologically:
- Enhanced sensory stimulation leads to decreased perception of pain.
- Restores normal muscle activation and function.
- Reinforces the restoration of functional stability.

- Promotes peripheral neuroplasticity.

- Stimulates the skin's endogenous analgesic system.

3. Improved microcirculatory function:

- produces pressure changes under the skin, thereby opening up channels to reduce and wash away injury and inflammation

- improved lymphatic flow

- improved superficial microcirculatory flow and better healing

The end result is improved performance and better prognosis for athletes. The athlete is able to perform daily activities without fearing pain or re-injury.

McConnell patellar taping:

McConnell is one of the most commonly used taping techniques to treat patellofemoral pain.

It was first introduced in 1984 by Jenny McConnell and since then has gradually become one of the most-preferred forms of treatment for patellofemoral pain.

Athletes and sedentary people often suffer from pain in the patella or kneecap. Anterior knee pain can be produced by many factors, which include tightness of tendons and muscles around the knee, abnormal movement of the kneecap during training and exercise, and direct injury to the kneecap during sport.

The usual mode of therapy for people suffering with kneecap pain includes physical therapy and rehabilitation. Along with the traditional treatment techniques, McConnell taping may be used to accelerate recovery and reduce pain in the kneecap.

The technique works on the premise of altering the tilt and position of the patella; this is achieved by shifting a laterally displaced patella more medially to correct patellofemoral "tracking" problems.

Many studies have been conducted to study the efficiency of the patellar taping technique; data from these studies shows that the taping technique produces altered patella kinematics, enhanced EMG and muscle function, improved dynamic alignment, and decreased patellofemoral joint-reaction forces.

While there is positive evidence from scientific studies to support the efficiency of the patellar taping technique, many experts debate about the effectiveness of these techniques and wait for conclusive evidence to be produced by more studies—however, most of them unanimously agree that the patellar taping technique decreases pain in subjects with patellofemoral injury.

How to use McConnell taping:

During the examination the patient is asked to flex/stretch the knee joint and patella, while the health care professional examines the location of the patella—this examination process is known as tracking. The subject may also be asked to perform common maneuvers such as squatting or walking up the stairs, and at the end of the physical movement the athlete is asked to rate the pain experienced during the physical movement.

An abnormal positioning or tracking indicates that there are tight tissues around the thigh that are pulling the kneecap toward the outside of the knee—the knee taping can prove to be useful in realigning the kneecap in such situations.

One of the greatest benefits of the patellar taping method is that it is fairly easy to learn, and the taping technique can be taught to another person within ten to fifteen minutes.

Many variations of the taping technique are available; therefore, the health-care professional may choose the taping technique according to the athlete's requirements. Since patellar taping provides quick pain relief, it allows the athlete to train with greater intensity.

There are two components to patellar taping:

1. White protective tape (Cover-Roll): the white tape adheres well to a non-oiled smoothly shaven surface—the white tape serves as a firm surface for a more-adhesive brown tape.

b) Brown tape: the brown tape has a strong adhesive surface and should not be applied directly to the skin. It acts as a firm tape and helps in pain reduction.

Note: Patellar taping in the lateral-to-medial direction will cause a medial shift in the patella for those that are laterally displaced; however, it produces just the opposite effect in people who have a medially displaced patella (i.e., the patella will actually move against the direction of taping). Taping is meant only to be a temporary treatment for knee pain; it should never be used as a substitute for physiotherapy and sports rehabilitation.

Specific proprioceptive response taping (SPRT):

SPRT was developed by Dr. Tim Brown and utilizes a variety of different tape types (Leukotape, Hypafix, Kinesio tape). SPRT taping helps determines the direction necessary for proper approximation and compression of injured tissues.

SPRT gives relief of the injury during movement through improving proprioception and neuromuscular control. Due to the types of tapes used, SPRT is very supportive of injured or torn tissues while still allowing for proper range of motion with activity. SPRT can be applied to a number of injuries, including the following:

1) Cervical and lumbar disc herniations (neck and lumbar disc injuries)

2) Shoulder/rotator cuff injuries

3) AC joint injuries (shoulder separations)

4) Tennis/golfer's elbow

5) Postural disorders

6) Knee tracking disorders (patella tracking disorders)

7) Ankle sprains

8) Meniscal injuries

Athletic or sport taping:

Athletic taping is a type of strapping technique that uses a white, rigid tape attached to the skin designed to physically support unstable joints, ligaments, and fascia. The intent of sports taping is to reduce pain, speed recovery from injury, and allow for continued participation in sport or recreation. Taping is typically used to help the athlete recover from acute- (ankle sprains) and overuse- (plantar fasciopathy) type injuries.

Physical therapy/physiotherapy:

- Physiotherapy: E-stim, Ultrasound, ice/heat, traction, Class III and Class IV laser, compression

Physiotherapy:

Electrical stimulation (E-stim):

E-stim is a modality of treatment that uses electrical current to produce a favorable effect on the tissue being treated. Electrical stimulation is commonly used to treat conditions such as pain, inflammation, muscle spasms, healing skin incisions, healing bone fractures, muscle atrophy, and improving delivery of medication through the skin. There are many forms of electrical stimulation: inferential, Russian, pre-mod, direct current, and microcurrent, to name a few. Each form has its area of optimal performance, and a qualified provided can use any of its forms.

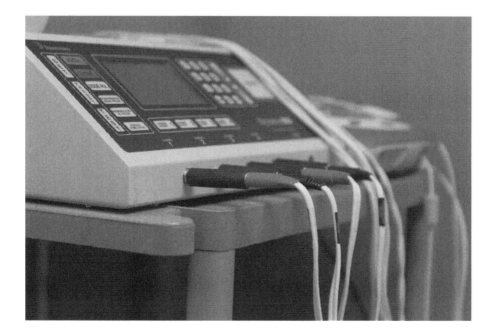

Electrical stimulation produces many favorable effects on the skin/muscles/ and joint tissues:

- stimulating muscles to contract

- stimulating nerves to decrease pain

- increasing blood flow to speed healing and reduce inflammation

- stimulating cells to reproduce and speed healing

- improving the flow of medication through the skin

- decreasing scar-tissue formation

- TENS units (the small units you can buy and use at home) are not the same and are solely used for pain control)

Ultrasound therapy in sports:

Ultrasound waves can strike muscle tissue at frequencies of a million times per second.

The ultrasound waves produce vibrations in the tendons and soft tissues; this produces a healing effect and helps in soothing the inflammation and pain in the area. The relaxation produced in the tendons and tissues facilitates better blood flow and reduces swelling and chronic inflammation.

Ultrasound is also known to improve the blood flow, thus facilitating better delivery of oxygen and nutrients to tissues and washing away cell waste more efficiently.

Mechanism of action:

Ultrasound therapy uses a frequency range of 0.9 to 3.0 MHz.

Ultrasound promotes healing in both the inflammatory and proliferative stages of wound resolution. Ultrasound exerts its effects by causing a degranulation of mast cells and triggering a release of histamine. The histamine produced further triggers the migration of neutrophils and monocytes to the injury site—this phenomenon improves the healing rate in injured and inflamed tissues.

Ultrasound is used for the following purposes in sports medicine:

- to break scar tissue and adhesions

- to reduce inflammation, swelling, and calcium deposits

- to reduce muscle spasms by creating heat in the localized area

- to increase soft-tissue extensibility prior to stretching and exercise

- to promote healing at the cellular level

- to speed up metabolism and improve blood flow

- to reduce nerve-root irritation

- to speed up bone healing

Heat and ice therapy for athletes:

Soft-tissues injuries and strain in the lower limbs can be treated through the use of alternating ice and heat therapy. This is especially useful in facilitating effective recovery after a long run, heavy workout, or acute soft-tissue injury.

Using heat and ice helps in producing a pumping mechanism that facilitates vasodilation with heat (opening up of blood vessels) and vasoconstriction with ice (closing up of blood vessels).

Heat helps in improving blood circulation and blood flow in the area, whereas ice helps in flushing out lactic acid and reduces soreness after workout.

The effect can be achieved through the use of hot and cold *baths* or through the application of hot and cold *packs*. There are many protocols that are used, depending on the athlete's condition.

Example of one protocol is as follows:

- 10 min ice followed 10 min heat;

- 8 min ice then 8 min heat;

- 6 min ice then 6 min heat;

- 4 min ice then 4 min heat;

- 2 min ice then 2 min heat; and

- end with 1–2 min of ice.

Home/field/locker-room care:

- Hot/cold: tubs and baths

Traction in sports medicine [7, 8, 9, 10]:

Traction therapy helps in reducing the pain that originates from the discs of the spine, and it addresses both the mechanical and function aspects of disc pain.

The amount of treatment required for higher levels of spinal retraction and disc rehydration can be calculated using computerized systems that will appropriately increase the amount of axial decompression. Spinal decompression works by creating a negative pressure within the disc—this helps the protruded or herniated disc material to be pushed back into the normal confines of the disc, thereby facilitating healing and recovery.

This procedure allows the pressure to be removed from the inflamed nerve roots, thus allowing the inflammation to subside and healing to occur.

Methodology:

The treatment provider determines the amount of force needed to gently stretch the bones of the lower back and neck; the negative pressure allows for the disc herniation to subside and improves the hydration status and promotes healing in the disc. The position of the traction pull and the height of the table can be adjusted; this helps the health-care professional to work on a particular segment of the spine and in a specific direction.

The treatment is painless; it also has the potential to produce immediate pain relief (due to decompression). The physiotherapist will use a combination of home exercises, decompression, and stabilization to achieve optimal results.

Traction is used to treat the following:

- bulging, prolapsed, or herniated discs

- spinal stenosis

- sciatica

- Facet syndrome

- degenerative disc disease

- neck pain

- pain radiating down the arm

- "pinched nerves"

- spondylitis

Nonsurgical Decompression:

Nonsurgical decompression is similar to traction; the equipments used in nonsurgical decompression are different and often more advanced than those used in traction therapy.

Disc injuries in the neck and low back are increasingly being treated with nonsurgical spinal decompression. This treatment option is considered to be safe and utilizes FDA-cleared equipment to apply distraction forces to spinal structures in a precise and graduated manner. The distraction is applied in cycles of partial relaxation.

Spinal decompression therapy works by gently separating the vertebrae from each other, creating a vacuum inside the discs that we are targeting. This vacuum effect is also known as negative intra-discal pressure.

The negative pressure may induce the retraction of the herniated or bulging disc into the inside of the disc, and off the nerve root, thecal sac, or both. It happens only microscopically each time, but cumulatively, over four to six weeks, the results are quite dramatic.

The cycles of decompression and partial relaxation, over a series of visits, promote the diffusion of water, oxygen, and nutrient-rich fluids from the outside of the discs to the inside. These nutrients enable the torn and degenerated disc fibers to begin to heal.

Compression therapy and its role in sports medicine:

Over the last few years, compression therapy has gained acceptance in the sporting world as a genuine means of improving sporting performance and post-event muscle recovery. Compression stockings are a widely used for compression therapy; many famous athletes use compression stockings in both their upper and lower extremities to facilitate better blood flow. Compression therapy works on the premise that increased venous return and blood flow should aid in the clearance of metabolic by-products such as lactate, which builds up during muscle exertion.

Increased blood flow and metabolite clearance in turn helps in improving recovery time and athletic performance.

ICE and compression:

<u>Game Ready:</u>

Game Ready combines intermittent compression with circumferential cold therapy in one adjustable system.

- Game Ready® uses ACCEL™ technology that synergistically combines active pneumatic compression and rapidly circulating cold therapy to do more than passively treat symptoms of pain and swelling. ACCEL creates the therapeutic power to accelerate the body's natural repair mechanisms by enhancing lymphatic function, encouraging oxygenated blood flow and stimulating tissue healing.

- Game Ready technology enables deeper, longer-lasting cold therapy. In addition, most other cold therapy does not offer compression—and if it does, it's usually static. While static compression is commonly accepted as a useful method for passively mitigating swelling, it does not help the body heal. By contrast, Game Ready's form of active compression mimics natural muscle contractions to stimulate tissue healing.

More information can be found at http://www.gameready.com.

Professional compression devices:

Recovery Boots:

Pneumatic medicine is the use of noninvasive, dynamic pneumatic compression to treat a variety of medical conditions associated with compromised peripheral circulation, including chronic wounds or ulcers, venous insufficiency, and lymphedema. Now teams are using them for recovery.

RecoveryPump delivers medical grade compression to help rid the muscle of fatigue, soreness, and inflammation.

Benefits:

1) Temporarily increases venous return/flow in the veins—it is intended to temporarily relieve muscle aches and pain and to temporarily increase circulation to the treated area after exercise.

2) Massaging action—a noninvasive intermittent sequential external pneumatic compression system that simulates kneading and stroking of tissues with the hands by use of an inflatable pressure cuff.

3) Reduces swelling—temporarily reduce swelling after muscle stress or injury.

When to use:

Post-exercise:

- Use as soon as possible after workout; this will reduce the window period available for soreness and fatigue to set in.

- Use thirty to forty-five minutes immediately after workout.

- Use at the end of the day after workout, job, family time, etc. for one to two hours or as needed.

How to use:

Set the PRESSURE to comfort level—60 mmHg is the standard setting; you may adjust increase or decrease the pressure as desired for comfort.

The standard setting for PAUSE time is ten seconds; if there are no sensory changes during the therapy session, the pause time may be increased to thirty seconds if sensation changes are felt in the foot or ankle area (pins and needles, pain, or numbness). If the sensation changes persist, stop pumping and see your doctor.

The therapy may be used more than once per day for recovery.

Use Recovery Pump® at least twice per day post-race for one to two hours per session for two to three days or until fully back into training program.

If you wish to sleep with the Recovery Pump®, increase the pause time to thirty to forty-five seconds. This will allow significantly more arterial flow to the extremities (a good thing, as the blood will be delivering lots of O2, H20, and nutrients). More information can be found at www. recoverypump.com.

Compression clothing:

Compression garments can help athletes in many different ways: skin protection, moisture wicking, increased performance, lower fatigue during travel, and improved rates of recovery.

Heavy training can often cause muscle soreness and posture strain; research studies have shown that compression clothing can be effective in minimizing swelling and improving the alignment and mobility.

Compression clothing works by allowing the arteriole walls to relax and increasing oxygen-rich blood flow (40 percent in some studies). In addition, graduated compression helps bring back deoxygenated blood to the heart.

Posture correction clothing:

IntelliSkin:

IntelliSkin provides therapeutic shirts, providing supportive compression and an aggressive PostureCue of the muscles that support and align the spine and shoulders. This shirt is ideal for athletes seeking the strongest posture improvement during workouts, recovery, running, and such sports as football and baseball.

<u>Benefits:</u>

- instantly feel taller, leaner, and stronger

- improved spinal alignment and posture

- increased mobility, stability, muscular balance, and stability

- better respiration, with increased circulation and oxygen flow to the brain and muscles, increasing endurance and reducing fatigue

- quicker recovery from training, competition, injury, and even traveling

- supports and enhances the rehabilitation process when treating injuries (wearing IntelliSkin after treatment can extend the benefits of that treatment)

- improved movement patterns through proper alignment and posture

- reduces the risk of injury associated with poor posture and repetitive movement patterns

Laser therapy in sports medicine:

What is laser therapy?

The concept of laser therapy was first theorized by Einstein in 1916; the technology for producing lasers came into existence since 1965. Laser therapy has since been used in many fields of science, and the medical community has made extensive use of laser for various therapeutic purposes.

How does it work?

Our bodies' tissues react to certain wavelengths of light by showing physiological responses and reactions. Laser exerts the following effects on the human body:

1) Oxygenated hemoglobin HbO2 can be deoxygenated by absorption of photon of radiation. Peak occurs at 970 nm.

2) The terminal enzyme in the respiratory chain of a cell is cytochrome C oxidase; this photo-absorber controls the rate at which oxygen is processed in the ATP of the mitochondria. An 800 nm beam of light influences cytochrome C function.

Laser can biostimulate the damaged tissues and help them heal faster and get stronger. Laser stimulates tissue regeneration and reduces inflammation and associated pain. Laser has many more benefits. Laser can be used to achieve the following list of therapeutic effects:

- decreased pain levels

- reduced inflammation

- increased tissue proliferation and regeneration

- accelerated soft-tissue and bone repair

- increased tissue tensile strength

- enhanced nerve regeneration and function

- increased cell metabolism

- increased enzymatic responses

- increased cell-membrane potentials

- increased microcirculation and vasodilation

- increased lymphatic flow

- increased collagen production

- enhanced angiogenesis (production of new blood vessels)

Types of laser:

There are two basic types of lasers: namely, hot lasers (class IV) and cold lasers (class III).

Hot lasers are mainly used in surgery; they help in cutting through the tissue. They are called hot lasers because they produce heat and burn the tissue they come in contact with.

Cold lasers/ Low-level lasers: These lasers generate laser light but do not generate heat. A cold laser maybe visible or invisible, depending on the chosen type and intensity. The cold lasers are not "cold," but they don't get hot either. Cold lasers are mostly used for their therapeutic purposes; they are often used to increase the rate of healing in damaged tissues, to increase blood flow, and to reduce infection.

Side effects of lasers:

Cold lasers don't have any reported side effects; however, caution should be used while handling lasers; if the lasers are projected directly into the eye, they can cause permanent damage to the retina; for this reason the health-care professional is advised to wear protective goggles.

- Lasers should not be used over the thyroid gland (neck area), since they can affect the rate of thyroid hormone production.

- Laser should not be used over a developing baby during pregnancy.

- Laser should not be used over cancerous growths, since it can increase the rate of cell multiplication and increase the rate of cancer growth.

Lasers are divided into four classes, depending upon the power or energy of the beam and the wavelength of the emitted radiation. Laser classification is based on the laser's potential for causing immediate injury to the eye or skin and/or potential for causing fires from direct exposure to the beam or from reflections from diffuse reflective surfaces. Since August 1, 1976, commercially produced lasers have been classified and identified by labels affixed to the laser.

Look for these labels on the laser product:

Class I:

- Inherently safe with no possibility of eye damage—this can be either because of a low output power (in which case eye damage is impossible even after hours of exposure), or due to an enclosure preventing user access to the laser beam during normal operation, such as in CD players or laser printers.

Class II:

- The blink reflex of the human eye (aversion response) will prevent eye damage, unless the person deliberately stares into the beam for an extended period. Output power may be up to 1 mW. This class includes only lasers that emit visible light. Some laser pointers are in this category.

Class IIa:

- A region in the low-power end of Class II, where the laser requires in excess of one thousand seconds of continuous viewing to produce a burn to the retina. Commercial laser scanners are in this subclass.

Class IIIa:

- Lasers in this class are mostly dangerous in combination with optical instruments that change the beam diameter or power density, though even without optical instrument, enhancement direct contact with the eye for over two minutes may cause serious damage to the retina. Output power does not exceed 5 mW. Beam power density may not exceed 2.5 mW/square cm. Many laser sights for fire-arms and laser pointers are in this category.

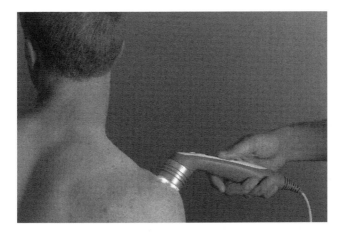

Class IIIb:

- Lasers in this class may cause damage if the beam enters the eye directly. This generally applies to lasers powered from 5–500 mW. Lasers in this category can cause permanent eye damage with exposures of 1/100th of a second or less, depending on the strength of the laser. A diffuse reflection is generally not hazardous, but reflections can be just as dangerous as direct exposures. Protective eyewear is recommended when direct beam viewing of Class IIIb lasers may occur. Lasers at the high power end of this class may also present a fire hazard and can lightly burn skin. A few "laser pointers" at 300 mW visible green output are now available in this category.

Class IV:

- Lasers in this class have output powers of more than 500 mW in the beam and may cause severe, permanent damage to eye or skin without being magnified by optics of eye or instrumentation. Diffuse reflections of the laser beam can be hazardous to skin or eye within the Nominal Hazard Zone. Most industrial, scientific, military, and medical lasers are in this category.

Types of lasers available in the market:

Low-level laser/Class III/cold laser:
- Low-level laser therapy began in 1967, after the experiments conducted by Endre Mester in Semmelweis University, Hungary, which showed many therapeutic benefits.

Commercially available laser:
- Erchonia: (Class IV) 5 milli watt; wavelength: 635 nm; Class IIIb—in January of 2002, Erchonia was the first low-level laser given market clearance by the Food and Drug Administration.

- K-laser: The K-Series Class IV therapy laser has power adjustable from 0.1 to 8 watts in the K-800 model, and 0.1 to 12 watts in the K-1200. The adjustable power allows for a wide range of treatment protocols. Class IV laser therapy delivers a therapeutic dosage to a large volume of tissue in a shorter period of time. The K-Series has dual 800 and 970 nm wavelength select ability.

- Cutting Edge Technologies MLS (http://med.celasers.com/): Class IV laser with a peak power of 25 watts; both the 808 nm and 905 nm wavelengths delivered simultaneously. The 808 nm wavelength is delivered using continuous emission, while the 905 nm wavelength is delivered using pulsed emission.

Self-massage for sports professionals:

Massage has numerous benefits for athletes: it helps improve blood circulation, and it reduces blood congestion and muscle stiffness. Research has also shown that massage can help in improving the athlete by stimulating the production of white blood cells. The physical effects of massage are welcome by people of all age groups; massage produces relaxation and relieves stress.

Athletes can benefit from regular massage; however, the athlete may not be able to hire a massage therapist on a regular basis due to a time crunch, extensive travel, or due to the unavailability/expense associated with good massage therapists.

The good news is that if you can't afford it, you don't need to hire a massage therapist; there are many efficient tools available in the market that can give a good massage experience and relieve muscle tension. Let's have a look at some of the most efficient methods of self-massage:

Hammering/tapping:

This exercise is known as "Mountain energy exercise" in Tai Chi and is known to reactivate the blood circulation and energy in the body. For this exercise, you will need to use your hands or a flat object to pat different parts of the body.

Many practitioners use a cupped palm or a fist to gently tap or thump various parts of the body in a systematic manner. Start patting/thumping from your feet and work your way upward. Then tap over your abdomen in a circular manner, gradually moving up to the upper limbs, neck, and head. Continue until you feel fully fresh and awake.

This exercise can be done both in the morning and the evening; it helps stimulate blood circulation and awakens the nerve endings.

Foam roller:

The foam roller is a cylindrical piece of hard-celled foam. It has a dense consistency and a large diameter; it is usually one to three feet in length. The foam roller is also available in many different densities, from very soft foam to hard, dense varieties. A heavyweight athlete with more body density should choose a denser foam roller, whereas a lighter athlete may choose a softer variety of foam.

The foam roller works on the principle of acupressure; the pressure is exerted on parts of the body that are strained. The athletes are asked to use the foam roller on the sensitive areas of their bodies that are prone to fatigue; these areas are known as trigger points or knots, and they have increased muscle density.

The athlete is asked to make a note of the injury-prone areas and to apply pressure to these areas on a regular basis using a foam roller. Most athletes are able to identify the tension spots on their own; these spots are usually tender and should be worked on until the density of the area decreases and the muscle group relaxes.

It is important to note that positioning the roller at different angles may produces different effects; the roller may be used in a parallel, perpendicular, or a forty-five-degree position, depending on the muscle. Factors such as age, fitness level, and comfort level should be considered while choosing the type of roller and the intensity of rolling.

The foam roller may also be used as a massager, and longer sweeping strokes may be used on large muscle groups such as calves, adductors, quadriceps, hip rotators, and gluteus medius.

The foam roller may be used at different times of the day for different purposes; the most commonly followed protocol is to use the roller before and after the exercise. Using a foam roller prior to the exercise helps reduce the muscle density and promotes a better warm-up; using the roller after the exercise will reduce the time required for recovery.

The foam roller can be used on any part of the body; however, it may be most beneficial to use the foam roller on the lower limbs, because they have a lot of muscle and tendon tissue; the upper limbs don't have dense muscle tissue; therefore, the athlete may not experience the same amount of benefit while using the foam roller on the upper limbs.

Trigger Point:

Trigger Point (TP) specializes in creating massage products that simulate the feeling of a human hand. They offer various tools such as the massage ball, TP quadballer, and various types of massage kits.

TP massage ball's primary focus is to assist in managing minor aches and pains of the muscle by applying pressure to general areas. Apply pressure with the ball by using the floor, wall, or any hard surface to stabilize movement of the ball. Understand that in order to get deep into the muscle, the ball has to remain still with an ample amount pressure for five to seven seconds. This is when the ball will change shape. Once relieved, roll the TP massage ball side to side or in circles for a cross-friction type of massage. The TP massage ball is great for the neck, shoulders, back, chest, piriformis, calves, or anywhere that you have minor aches and pains.

The TP quadballer allows you to roll completely through the quads, IT band, lower back, hamstrings, and neck in a safe and effective manner.

More information and videos about these tools can be found at http://www.tptherapy.com/.

Self cross friction massage:

This massage is most effective for treating tendonitis (inflammation of the tendon that connects the muscle to the bone); it works on the premise of "scrubbing" the fibers instead of a deep, intense massage; it is believed that mild stimulation often speeds up natural tissue repair mechanisms in the tendons. The method has no side effects and is easy to try, even for beginners.

How to do the massage:

The massage technique is fairly straightforward and simple. Locate the greatest point of tenderness in the muscle/tendon and rub the area gently back and forth over the inflamed area—the direction of your massage strokes must be perpendicular to the fibers of the tendon you're working on. This is identical to rubbing the strings of a guitar; i.e., imagine that the tender point is a taut string; your massage will help relieve the tension and speed up recovery.

Use the pads of your fingers or the thumb and apply gentle pressure to work on the area; there is no need for strong pressure in this type of massage.

Expect discomfort during the massage; the pain may be sharp or may cause a burning sensation; if the friction doesn't produce any pain, then you are probably massaging the wrong place.

Any discomfort you experience during this massage will subside within a couple of minutes; if the pain doesn't stop, then you may choose to stop the treatment and try it again later.

If the pain is too intense, even though the pressure you are exerting is minimal, then it means that the tendonitis you are experiencing is serious, and you probably need medical attention.

Recommended procedure:

- Use friction massage for one to two minutes, until sensitivity in the region subsides.

- Increase the intensity slightly. Use friction for one to two minutes, until sensitivity subsides.

- Increase the intensity slightly more. Use friction for one to two minutes, until sensitivity subsides.

You may finish the massage by applying bare ice on the site. (Apply the ice for about two to three minutes on the spot or until the area becomes numb; whichever is earlier.) You should be able to complete the full massage routine within three to six minutes.

You may choose to do the massage for up to three times a day—if the pain you are experiencing comes from tendonitis, then you should feel an immediate relief from symptoms.

The stick massage:

The stick is a widely used massage tool than can improve flexibility and promote muscle recovery.

The stick works by simultaneously compressing, stretching, and warming the muscle, facilitating myofascial release, inactivating trigger points (muscle knots/kinks), and increasing circulation. During the process you will feel the muscle knots that are hindering your performance, and these muscle knots will slowly disappear with the massage.

The massage promotes fresh blood flow and increases the quality of the connective tissue in the region—this process helps the body and muscle groups to regenerate, and this in turn results in better mobility, faster muscle recovery, additional strength, and lowered chances of injury.

When to use the massage stick:

The massage stick maybe used during the *pre-exercise period* to promote muscle warm-up and to ensure maximum flexibility during the training session.

The massage stick maybe used during the *post-exercise period* to relax the muscles, promote blood flow, and improve muscle recovery.

It may also be used early in the morning or just before bed to relax and rejuvenate.

Benefits of stick massage:

Tight muscles—removes trigger points, allowing the muscle to relax and recover.

Muscle injury—improves flexibility and blood circulation, which greatly reduces the incidence of injury, and, if injury does occur, assists the natural healing and recovery process.

Calf muscles, hamstrings, ITBS, back, neck, and forearms can easily be treated with the stick. The easy rolling action gently massages away your muscle problems.

Altitude tents:

An altitude tent helps simulate an environment of high altitude. Our red blood cells are vital for muscle function; they help in carrying oxygen to various tissues in the body. By living or training in an altitude tent, the athlete has the opportunity to adapt to an environment with lower oxygen content—this is particularly beneficial, because, when the body experiences high-altitude conditions, it starts producing more red blood cells and hemoglobin, which are capable of carrying oxygen.

The body achieves many positive adaptations when it's exposed to high-altitude environments; the high-altitude tent also provides an additional benefit—athletes can still practice at the gym in a normal oxygen environment during the day, and their bodies produce more blood cells in the high-altitude tent during sleep at night.

Needless to say that the athlete will benefit enormously by the improved supply of oxygen to the tissues; such small differences in metabolism can give the athlete the winning edge.

Mechanism of action:

High-altitude environments typically have low air pressure—this environment is difficult to produce in an indoor setting, because it would require use of an airlock to prevent implosion and significant engineering; for this reason the tent uses a different technology to produce a high-altitude environment; it uses a special device to bring down the oxygen content inside: the normal air contains about 20.9 percent oxygen, while the air in the altitude tent is adjusted to 12 percent oxygen.

Most altitude tents use a machine known as the hypoxic air generator, which pumps hypoxic air into the tent. The general simulation setting used by most athletes inside altitude tents is between 8,000 and 15,000 ft. A significant physiological response is produced by the athlete's body only when the body's oxygen saturation content drops below 90 percent.

Under such a hypoxic state, the body strives to make more efficient use of the oxygen available and starts producing a protein known as hypoxia inducible factor (HIF-1) to improve its capacity to use oxygen.

Altitude tents produce the following physiological reactions:

1) Increased oxygen absorption in the pulmonary space.

2) Increased production of erythropoietin hormone (EPO) by the kidneys, which in turn stimulates the generation of red blood cells (RBCs) and enhances oxygen transport throughout the body.

3) Increase in number of capillaries—this in turn provides better oxygen supply to muscles, tissues, and brain cells.

4) Improved production and regeneration of mitochondria and related enzymes—this helps in increasing the levels of energy and provides superior enzymatic antioxidative defense.

5) Decreased heart rate.

6) Reduced blood pressure.

7) Improved production of human growth hormone.

8) Better rate of fat metabolism.

9) Reduced rate of oxidative stress from free radicals.

Different types of high-altitude systems:

Altitude sleeping systems—these systems are meant for professional athletes looking to boost their performance with a "sleep-high, train-low" training regimen or for the mountaineer looking to maximize exposure to high altitude for purposes of pre-acclimatization.

Altitude workout systems—These systems help you burn off a few extra calories by adding altitude workouts to your training. These mask-based systems are perfect for home use in conjunction with an individual's exercise equipment of choice. Benefits can be noticed by professional athletes as well as amateur athletes within a few days of training.

Floatation tanks:

Research studies conducted on human physiology show that most of the energy consumed by the brain's normal workload is due to presence of environmental elements such as gravity, variable temperature, touch, and effects of light, sound and pressure on various systems in the body. Therefore, removing most of these elements will reduce the amount of energy spent by the body; this saved-up energy can then be used for faster recovery.

The floatation tank was designed specifically for this purpose; it removes all the external environmental stimuli and creates a state of complete sensory relaxation.

The tank usually contains water with Epsom salt, which gives the body buoyancy and helps it float on the liquid and has many healing properties.

The athlete relaxes and reclines backward; the athlete's ears are submerged below the solution; the athlete may choose silence or may listen to ambient music of choice—most floatation tanks come with an inbuilt underwater sound system that delivers high-quality music.

The temperature is maintained at a constant inside the floatation tank— usually 34.5 Celsius, which is the relaxed skin temperature. After a while the skin gets acclimatized to the surrounding liquid temperature, and the athlete may not perceive any sense of separation between his or her skin and the surrounding liquid; this gives a sensation of floatation.

With time, the athlete enters deeper levels of relaxation, and there is a significant decrease in brain activity. The relaxation can be compared to a stage of deep sleep, except that the athlete is awake. The quality of rest, rejuvenation, and recovery achieved by this method is very high.

Scientific studies on floatation tanks:

The effects of restricted environmental stimulation technique (REST) have been researched and documented at Stanford, Harvard, Yale, and countless other universities, hospitals, and sports-training facilities around the world. Professional and scientific work with float tanks is coordinated by a body called IRIS (International REST Investigators Society) in New York.

IRIS was founded in 1982.

Research papers presented at these conferences [11, 12, 13, and 14] have also been published in books. They have covered research topics such as the effects of floating on

- enhancement of creativity;

- improvement in sporting performance;

- stress management;

- biological effects;

- psycho/physiological effects;

- better hypnosis induction;

- skin disease;

- treatment of habit disorders;

- treatment of physical and psychological disorders, such as anxiety;

- relief from premenstrual syndrome (PMS);

- relief from chronic pain; and

- relief from rheumatoid arthritis.

For information on certain topics concerning the effects of floating, you may contact IRIS.

Oxygen tents:

The saturation of oxygen in blood plays a major role in the oxygen transport to tissues. Oxygen tents provide a 3 psi hyperbaric pressure, which increases the ambient environmental pressure from 760 mmHg (normal atmospheric pressure) to 915 mmHg.

Henry's Law states, "a gas is dissolved by a liquid in direct proportion to its partial pressure." For example, at sea level, atmospheric pressure is 760 mm Hg, the oxygen concentration is 21 percent, and the body's oxygen content or partial pressure, pO_2, in blood and plasma is around 40 mm Hg.

Typically the partial pressure of oxygen increases under such circumstances—this allows for more oxygen to be dissolved in a given unit of blood and helps increase the supply of oxygen to muscles.

Red blood cells have a limitation as to how much oxygen can bind with hemoglobin. The plasma portion of the blood typically has about a 3 percent oxygen concentration. This form of treatment can increase the amount of oxygen dissolved in plasma.

Such treatment is known as hyperbaric oxygen therapy (HBOT) and is recommended for increasing oxygen supply to tissues.

The changes produced in oxygen levels at 3 psi of atmospheric are significant; in fact, the amount of oxygen dissolved in the plasma is enough to help the athlete survive even in the absence of hemoglobin.

Six significant physiologic effects can be noted through hyperbaric therapy:

- reduction of volume of gas bubbles in the blood

- vasoconstriction, which reduces edema and secondary hypoxia

- decreased load on the heart

- restoration of aerobic metabolism to ischemic tissue

- detoxification of poisoned tissues

- enhanced phagocytosis

The most marked and important benefit for athletes is the increase in oxygen supply to lungs and tissues. It also eases respiratory symptoms such as cough and dried-up secretions that occur in respiratory conditions.

The subject must consult a doctor and get a complete physical checkup to rule out any conditions that can contraindicate the use of oxygen tents; special precautions must be taken for athletes with heart and lung diseases.

Physical medicine and surgery in sports medicine:

The common medications used in sports medicine include nonsteroidal anti-inflammatory drugs (NSAIDS), medications for pain (including opioids) and antispasmodic drugs.

A. NSAIDS:

The commonly used NSAIDS are ibuprofen, naproxen, fenoprofen, ketoprofen, flurbiprofen, oxaprozin, loxoprofen, aspirin (acetylsalicylic acid), and diflunisal salsalate.

The major side effect with NSAIDs is gastric discomfort; it was predicted that the advent of COX-2 inhibitors would reduce gastrointestinal discomfort; however, there is no substantial proof that COX-2 inhibitors reduce gastric symptoms or side effects.

The original study touted by Searle (now part of Pfizer), showing a reduced rate of ADRs for celecoxib, was later revealed to be based on preliminary data—the final data showed no significant difference in ADRs when compared with diclofenac.

Rofecoxib seemed to be a promising drug with very little gastric side-effect; however, concerns were raised regarding its cardiovascular study: the APPROVe trial, showed a statistically significant relative risk of cardiovascular events of 1.97 versus placebo—a result that prompted the worldwide withdrawal of rofecoxib in October 2004.

B. Other pain medications (includes opioids and narcotics):

These include codeine, oxycodone, hydrocodone, dihydromorphine, and pethidine.

C. Antispasmodics:

These include cyclobenzaprine, carisoprodol, orphenadrine, and tizanidine. Effectiveness has not been clearly shown for metaxalone, methocarbamol, chlorzoxazone, baclofen, or dantrolene. In a book called *Worst Pills, Best Pills II* by Sidney M. Wolfe et al., most of these medications were listed under DO NOT USE. I would have to agree and have found them to just be a central nervous system relaxer, and, when prescribed by some of my colleges, have left my athletes sleepy and dehydrated.

Medical therapy:

Platelet-rich plasma therapy (PRP):

Scientific studies have shown that wound and soft tissue healing are activated by platelet therapy.

PRP is an innovative method of relieving pain by promoting long-lasting healing; this technique has shown great potential for reducing the pain associated with musculoskeletal damage such as anterior cruciate ligament (ACL) injuries; rotator cuff tears; osteoarthritis of several joints, including hip, spine, shoulder and knee; pain and instability in the pelvis; chronic plantar fasciitis; tennis elbow, ankle sprains, tendonitis, and ligament sprains; and in back and neck injuries.

How does PRP therapy work?

The first response of the body to a soft-tissue injury is to deliver platelet cells to the affected site. Filled with growth and healing factors, the platelets begin the process of repair and also attract the vital aid of the body's stem cells. PRP therapy's completely natural healing process increases the body's efforts to heal by delivering a higher concentration of platelets to the site.

To produce PRP therapy, a small sample of the patient's blood is drawn (similar in amount to a sample for a lab test), which is then placed in a centrifuge to spin the blood at a high rate of speed to separate the platelets from the other blood components. This concentrated platelet-rich plasma (PRP) is then injected into the point of injury and surrounding tissue, thus jump-starting and significantly strengthening the body's natural ability to heal. Because the patient's own blood is used, there is no possible risk of infection being transmitted and also a very low risk of an allergic reaction.

Prolotherapy:

Proliferation therapy (or prolotherapy) has gained popularity in the medical community as an alternative treatment for chronic pain; it has been used in the treatment of different types of musculoskeletal pain, such as arthritis, back pain, neck pain, fibromyalgia, sports injuries, unresolved whiplash injuries, carpal tunnel syndrome, chronic tendonitis, partially torn tendons, ligaments and cartilage, degenerated or herniated discs, TMJ, and sciatica.

Prolotherapy treatments do not require invasive surgery to eliminate acute or chronic pain. Instead, prolotherapy offers a safe, effective treatment for patients interested in living a pain-free life without surgery.

Procedure:

Many solutions are used in prolotherapy; these include dextrose (a sugar), lidocaine (a commonly used local anesthetic), phenol, glycerin, or cod-liver-oil extract. The liquid is injected into joints or tendons where they connect to bone. The injected solution causes the body to heal itself through the process of inflammation and repair. The process may result in as much as 30–40 percent strengthening of the connective tissue.

For this reason, millions of prolotherapy injections are given each year by hundreds of physicians across the United States, and this technique has been adopted by many physicians across the world.

Uses of prolotherapy:

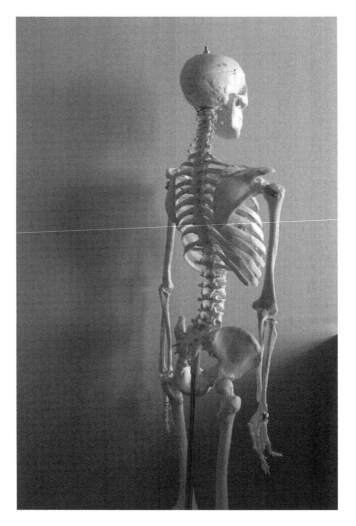

Prolotherapy may be used in the following cases:

- recurrent headache, face pain, jaw pain, ear pain

- chronic pain in joints

- chronic back pain

- chest pain with tenderness along the rib attachments on the spine or along the front of the chest

- spine pain that does not respond to surgery, or whose origin is not clear or consistent based on extensive studies

- recurrent swelling or fullness involving a joint or muscular region

- popping, clicking, grinding, or catching sensations with movement

- a sensation of the "leg giving way" with associated back pain

- temporary benefit from chiropractic manipulation or manual mobilization that fails to ultimately resolve the pain

- distinct tender points and "jump signs" along the bone at tendon or ligament attachments

- numbness, tingling, aching, or burning, referred into an upper or lower extremity

Other forms of injection therapies:

Hyaluronate (nonsulfated glycosaminoglycan) injection:

Hyalgan, Synvisc, Synvisc-One, and ORTHOVISC® are all viscosupplementation that can act as a shock absorber in the knee, with some studies showing improvement for up to six months.

Cortisone: injectable cortisone is synthetically produced and has many different trade names (e.g., Celestone and Kenalog).

Stem-cell therapy:

Stem-cell therapy is a fast-growing area of medicine. Stem cells have the potential to regenerate into to any type of tissue; they can repair damaged and injured cells.

Mechanism of action:

1) Stem cells themselves may be taken up by native tissue and then grow and multiply into new tissue.

2) Stem cells might secrete proteins that signal the native cells to multiply into new tissue.

Method:

Stem cells may be implanted in to the target tissue by a process known as microfracture surgery. In this procedure the doctor will drill holes in bone, so the marrow would leak out, and the stem cells would help heal various tissues (bone marrow stem cells).

Embryonic stem cells are more controversial in that they can potentially develop into anything (e.g., cancer cells).

Extracorporeal shockwave therapy (ESWT):

ESWT is a derivative of lithotripsy, the mechanical breaking up of renal stones with sound waves. Currently ESWT is approved for treatment of tennis elbow and plantar fasciitis. In the future, the FDA may approve ESWT therapy for treatment of specific ailments such as patella tendinitis, shoulder tendinitis, Achilles tendinitis, pseudoarthrosis, stress fractures, and shoulder calcification.

Mechanism of action:

Many theories have tried to explain the mechanism of action of ESWT; however, the most accepted view is that ESWT promotes healing by neovascularization (formation of new blood vessels) as a result of repeated micro-trauma caused by shockwaves. ESWT can even break down calcium deposits.

The new blood vessels increase the supply of nutrients and thereby promote better healing.

Another common theory is that the brain adapts to chronic presence of pain and ignores activity and healing in areas of chronic injury—ESWT creates a new inflammatory process and thereby activates the brain, which consequently sends new nutrients and other necessary substances to heal the area.

Method:

Completely noninvasive, it delivers sound waves in pulses from a device positioned at the injury site. It is the most advanced and highly effective noninvasive treatment method approved by the FDA. The procedure is performed in an outpatient setting; earlier it was performed under local anesthesia, taking up to thirty minutes. Now, with newer technology, it is possible to carry out the procedure without anesthesia at the physician's office in less than ten minutes.

The subject may require three to five sessions (not yet covered by insurance).

What disorders can be treated?

Generally acute or chronic muscle pain and/or tendon insertional pain:

- neck

- shoulder

- back and chest

- upper extremity

- lower extremity

- foot and ankle

- myofascial trigger points

Side effects:

There are no side effects associated with the therapy; the athlete may feel some form of pulse effect or discomfort at the site of treatment, but these effects are minor.

Recovery tools:

Restwise:

Restwise combines monitoring tools and software to create an accurate platform to measure the athlete's level of fatigue in response to training.

The device consists of a simple finger-clip pulse oximeter that measures the resting heart rate along with the oxygen saturation to give a clue about the body's metabolism.

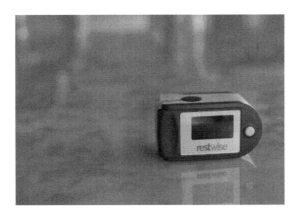

Restwise comes with web-based software that collects information about vital parameters such body weight, muscle soreness, and sleep duration; the software then runs its algorithm to give you a score that describes how fatigued your body is.

The pulse oximeter gives an instant reading, and answering the questionnaire takes about five minutes—such a system provides the athlete with real-time data and scores that allow him or her to avoid overtraining and monitor the daily levels of fatigue.

The questions probably provide more insight into the athlete's overall state of recovery than the pulse ox numbers give. However, the combination of all this data and its analysis is what Restwise is counting on to get you to your "recovery score."

Restwise markers include:

• resting heart rate	• energy level
• body mass	• mood stat
• sleep	• well-being
• oxygen saturation	• previous day's performance
• hydration	• rest
• appetite	• illness
• muscle soreness	

Zeo sleep manager uses a lightweight headband that tracks your actual sleep stages through the night and sends them wirelessly to your smartphone. This device has been described in detail in the *Sleep tools* section of this book.

Testing for oxidative stress:

Why is oxidative-stress-testing important?
The cells in our bodies are surrounded by a phospholipid membrane that is made up of fatty acids. Daily processes such as breathing produce substances known as free radicals, which are capable of causing damage to the phospholipid membrane; this process is described as oxidative stress.

Many diseases, as well as exposure to toxins, are known to cause oxidative stress; these can include heart disease, cancer, autoimmune and neurodegenerative diseases, rapid aging, and others (Trevisan 2001).

Revelar reagent test:

The Revelar reagent test measures a patient's baseline aldehyde level and provides a numerical score.

Aldehydes are the end product of a process that breaks down phospholipids via a chemical chain reaction that starts with the formation of unstable compounds known as lipid hydroperoxides and ends with aldehyde release. Numerous studies over the past three decades using tissue or plasma samples have shown that certain low-molecular-weight compound aldehydes are very effective biomarkers of oxidative stress.

The classic gold standard for measuring oxidative stress was the T-bar test; however, it has been widely criticized in large part because it measures a single aldehyde, MDA. Revelar measures multiple aldehydes, including important saturated aldehydes found in the gas phase of breath.

How it works:

The test measures the level of aldehydes in your breath. Studies show that aldehydes are direct by-products of oxidative stress. The higher the score shown by the test, the more aldehydes found in your breath, which may indicate higher oxidative stress. On a scale of one to one thousand, our range in "normal" subjects is between three hundred and nine hundred. The higher the score, the higher the aldehyde level.

After establishing a baseline, you have a starting point to understand your aldehyde levels and can take the steps to reduce those levels.

Tools to detect overtraining:

Heart-rate variability:

From beat to beat, your heart rate (HR) naturally increases and decreases in a cycle, known as HRV, or heart-rate variability.

It's been found that prolonged training leads to changes in autonomic cardiac balance. This sympathetic and parasympathetic balance can now be studied using HRV. Monitoring HRV provides a lot more insights than just plain heart-rate monitoring. It helps in assessing the effects of stress on the body.

Research studies [17] show that high HRV tends to represent good health and a high level of fitness, while decreased HRV is linked to stress, fatigue, and even burnout. Expert researchers have found that daily monitoring using standard HRV methods have shown that listening to your heart via HRV can not only stop you from overtraining but also can make your training more effective. [18]

Successful monitoring of HRV helps athletes to avoid severe overtraining and allows them to have a healthy recovery period.

Tools to measure HRV:

Polar OwnOptimizer is an easy and reliable way to determine whether your training program is optimally improving your performance.

Polar OwnOptimizer is a modification of a traditional orthostatic overtraining test. This equipment is based on heart rate and HRV measurements taken during an orthostatic test (standing up from relaxed resting).

OwnOptimizer helps you to optimize your training load during a training program, so that you do not undertrain or overtrain in the long run.

Polar OwnOptimizer is based on regular, long-term measurements of five heart-rate parameters. Two of these five values are calculated at rest, one while standing up, and two while standing. Each time you perform the test, the wrist unit saves the heart rate values and compares them to the previous values registered.

Baseline tests:

When you use OwnOptimizer for the first time, six baseline tests should be conducted over a period of two weeks to determine your personal baseline value. These baseline measurements should be taken during two typical basic training weeks, not during heavy training weeks. The baseline measurements should include tests taken after a training day and after recovery days.

Monitoring your OwnOptimizer values:

After the baseline recordings, you should continue to perform the test two to three times a week. Test yourself weekly in the morning following both a recovery day and a heavy training day (or a series of heavy training days).

An optional third test can be performed after a normal training day. OwnOptimizer may not provide reliable information during detraining or in a very irregular training period. If you take a break from exercise for fourteen days or longer, the baseline tests should be performed again.

The test checks to see how the nervous system controls the heart in response to different loads placed on it; in this case the load is that of simply lying down and standing up.

OwnOptimizer advises you about what state you are *currently* in. There are nine states ranging from "Good recovery" to "Parasympathetic over-training," and with each state you can get an idea about what to consider for your upcoming training.

Polars OwnIndex:

This is a fitness test using resting HR and HRV to provide an indication of oxygen uptake. The range of the OwnIndex is the same as that for VO2max, from 25 (which can be measured for unfit sedentary individuals) to 95 (which is the level reached by Olympic athletes such as top cross-country skiers).

VO2max is highest in sports, such as cross-country skiing and cycling, that involve large muscle groups. Fitness tests are most useful when following individual progress by comparing new results to previous ones.

For more information go to ww.polarusa.com.

Suunto uses EPOC (excess post-exercise oxygen consumption):

Our bodies consume excess oxygen during the recovery period after training; this excess amount of oxygen consumed during recovery is known as EPOC (excess post-exercise oxygen consumption).

EPOC is typically calculated from the HRV data, and therefore it is directly related to the physiological training load and accumulated cardiovascular fatigue; for this reason EPOC can be used to assess the training load on the athlete.

EPOC values increase with the intensity of the training: if the athlete exercises at low intensity for long stretches of time, then the EPOC value does not increase, but if the athlete trains at high intensity, the EPOC value increases considerably.

Many accurate and reliable devices are available to measure EPOC based on HR during exercise. This method has demonstrated remarkable precision, within 0.89 of traditional EPOC measurement.

Interpretation: a higher EPOC indicates insufficient recovery from previous sessions.

Benefits of measuring EPOC:

EPOC helps in studying the physical effects of an entire training session or a single workout.

- It is useful to assess the effects of any type of exercise at any intensity, with or without breaks.
- It educates you about your body's need for rest.

Training effect:

Another important parameter to monitor is the training effect (TE)—it is an accurate measurement of how hard the athlete has trained. A device known as the Suunto heart rate monitor helps in calculating the training effect; it uses data from your personal profile and combines it with a real-time analysis of your physiological progress. Your heart rate monitor then formulates your training effect and presents it on a scale from one to five.

Rest-Q sport:

Rest-Q is a tool that uses a questionnaire to help evaluating the athlete's recovery. Adequate recovery helps in restoring the body to its pre-exercise state and to prepare it for the next bout of exercise.

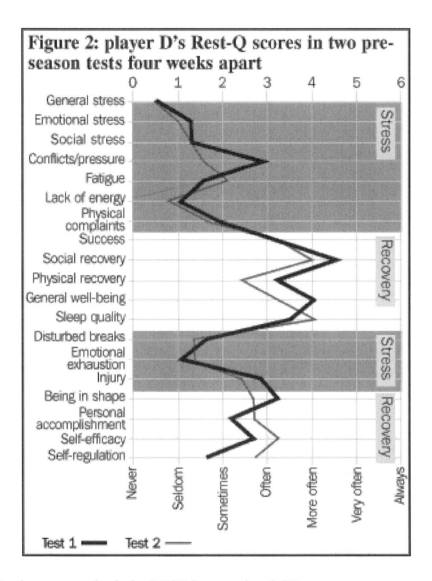

Figure 2: player D's Rest-Q scores in two pre-season tests four weeks apart

Equipment required: the RESTQ manual and CD, computer

Procedure: the RESTQ-Sport questionnaire measures stress and recovery rates in athletes. The manual gives the user the tools needed to measure and track an athlete's recovery.

The CD includes a database and scoring program. You are able to create a database of both individuals and groups. There are two questionnaires (RestQ-76 and Rest-52), scoring keys and profile sheets for the questionnaires.

Dartfish technology:

Dartfish technology is designed to easily integrate video during training and give athletes instant visual feedback, thus making it easier for them to understand the corrections and adjustments they need to make according to the trainer's inputs. This helps in improving and accelerating the learning process of athletes.

Dartfish Technology has been incorporated into multiple programs, including kinesiology, athletic training, sport management, physical education, athletics, and research.

Dartfish can be used as a bike fitting in cycling to assess cycling style and movement; it can be used to assess the gait of runners; and it allows the analyst to slow down the images and pinpoint the actions that could be causing trouble.

Dartfish allows you to

- use your expertise to enhance video images with its powerful analysis tools;

- highlight techniques and movements by selecting key moments on the video;

- compare them with reference clips, and use exclusive drawing and measurement tools;

- categorize your videos with personal attributes and create an index of events (e.g., serve, set, point); and

- easily retrieve specific actions from the index you created and make tactical and statistical analyses.

Functional movement assessment and/or screen:

There are many two main assessments that I like to use. The first one I became certified in was based on the National Academy of Sports Medicine corrective exercise specialist (CES).

National Academy of Sports Medicine CES:
Corrective exercise specialization: What is it?

A CES undergoes specialized training that teaches him or her to assess the neuromusculoskeletal balance in athletes during the training sessions and during the recovery phase after injury; the specialist is taught how to create a fully integrated conditioning program that takes place *prior* to mainstream strength and conditioning, or along with sports training as the required focus.

The CES studies human movement system (HMS), which is based on the concept that the body's muscle groups work as an integrated whole, with primary muscles, agonist and antagonist muscles, synergist muscles, and stabilizer muscles, all taking turns at various phases in time and during each motion of the human body.

What causes impairments in athletes:
1) The athlete may suffer from problems related to *poor posture*; the athlete's poor posture may be related to the exercise routine, sporting routine, or to normal daily activities such as working at a computer in a slouched position.

The specialist will make a note of the major activities the athlete performs throughout the day and will assess the postural orientation during these activities. The observation may be done in real time (at the spots gym) or in a simulated lab environment.

2) Poor rehabilitation: injury sustained by athletes can lead to restriction of activity and atrophy of associated muscles; if the injury is not followed up with an appropriate rehabilitation plan that aims to train all the atrophied muscles, then the athlete may never regain proper posture and movement after recovery; this leads to imbalance and reduced performance in sports. This is most often the case when an athlete complains of poor form after injury.

3) Sport-specific imbalance: The specialist will also asses if athletes' sporting requirements cause them to over-rely on certain muscle groups, thereby leading to hypertrophy of associated muscles—this phenomenon can disturb the overall muscular balance and affect the posture and performance of the athlete.

4) Incomplete rehabilitation: poor rehabilitation is not the only cause of muscular imbalance; if the athlete fails to follow a complete rehabilitation program, it can lead to muscular imbalance and reduced performance.

All the conditions mentioned above can lead to the development of compensation patterns, which have the potential to cause chronic joint and skeletal muscle problems.

Methodology:
The initial assessments of CES may include the following:

- static postural assessments

- functional movement testing

- range of motion testing

- muscle strength testing

The specialist will then create a conditioning program based on the integrated assessments; this program will allow the client to gain back the muscular balance and edge in athletic performance.

The assessments will be followed up with National Academy of Sports Medicine protocol for rehabilitation, which includes

- inhibition of overactive muscle/muscle groups;

- lengthening those muscles through SMR, static, and PNF stretching;

- activation techniques to progressively reeducate and strengthen weak (underactive and long) muscles; and lastly,

- integration techniques using progressively advanced, full-body exercises.

The CES program is highly active, and it helps the client work through all the above mentioned four phases until functional muscle balance is achieved; this process usually takes between four and eight weeks.

CES includes conditioning for the following ailments:

- foot and ankle impairments (including sprains and plantar fasciitis)

- low back pain (people sitting for more than three hours a day are at an increased risk of musculoskeletal degeneration due to poor posture)

- knee injuries (ACL injuries occur most often within the fifteen to twenty-five years of age group)

- shoulder injuries: shoulder impingement usually accounts for the greatest portion of diagnosis, and, if not dealt with, can lead to degenerative conditions of the shoulder structure, including rotator cuff issues.

The movement assessment consists of a series of full-body movement tests that assess the basic patterns of motion; these could include analysis of common movements such as bending and squatting in those with known musculoskeletal pain.

Such an assessment helps the health-care professional to identify the most dysfunctional non-painful movement pattern, which is then assessed in detail.

The health-care professional will then advise the athletes to make the necessary changes in posture, muscle balance, and the basic patterns of movement to facilitate better musculoskeletal motion.

By addressing the most dysfunctional non-painful pattern, the treatment (manual therapy and therapeutic exercise) is not disturbed by pain.

Recommended resources to learn functional movement assessment:

- National Academy of Sports Medicine: Functional Movement Assessment

- Gray Cooks: Selective Functional Movement Assessment (SFMA)

- Shirley A. Sahrmann: Two books on movement impairment syndromes

(Below) Photos from functional movement assessment: Knees Move Inward

Musculoskeletal diagnostic ultrasound:

Musculoskeletal ultrasound (MSK ultrasound) is a dynamic, noninvasive exam that allows high-resolution, real-time evaluation of musculoskeletal disorders. It is an excellent complement to MRI and a reliable modality for diagnosing musculoskeletal disorders related to traumatic injury, degeneration, and for patients who can't undergo MRI.

Noninvasive and dynamic imaging is beneficial when range of motion is lost due to acute or chronic injury to major tendons, as well as in pain management and urgent care. Musculoskeletal ultrasound is a unique modality that will enhance patient care.

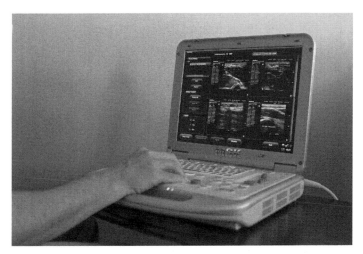

Diagnostic ultrasound capabilities:

What MSK ultrasound can be used for:
- shoulder examination: evaluation of shoulder pain or dysfunction

- elbow examination: soft-tissue injury, tendon pathology (including tendinopathy, enthesopathy, and tears), ligament pathology, arthritis, loose bodies, soft-tissue masses, nerve entrapment, effusion, and bone injury

- wrist and hand examination: soft-tissue injury, tendon pathology (tendinopathy, tenosynovitis, and tears), arthritis, soft-tissue masses or swelling (including ganglion cysts), nerve entrapment, effusion, foreign bodies, and bone injury

- hip examination: soft-tissue injury, tendon pathology, arthritis, soft-tissue masses or swelling, nerve entrapment, effusion, and bone injury

- knee examination: soft-tissue injury, tendon and collateral ligament pathology, arthritis, soft-tissue masses or swelling, loose intra-articular bodies, effusion, and bone injury

- ankle and foot examination: soft-tissue, tendon, and ligament injury; arthritis; soft-tissue masses or swelling; intra-articular loose bodies; effusion; bone injury; Morton's neuroma; plantar fasciitis; stress fracture; and foreign bodies

- peripheral nerve examination: compression neuropathies, neuritis, nerve masses, nerve trauma, and nerve subluxation

OmegaWave:

With the OmegaWave athletic training system, you can measure the athlete's cardiac fatigue, stress level, and adaptation reserves in just two minutes at rest. Training advice, recovery guidelines, and overall trends are sent directly to your smart device. This helps the athlete train smarter.

How it works:

In two minutes at rest, the OmegaWave ECG sensor belt measures and records data that assesses the athlete's readiness to train.

The OmegaWave software application then provides training advice, recovery guidelines, suggests aerobic and anaerobic thresholds, and reflects trends regarding your overall aerobic condition.

The OmegaWave system helps optimize every training session. It gives important clues on when the athlete can train hard and when the athlete needs to rest.

The device provides important clues into the following systems:

- cardiac system

- energy metabolism

- neuromuscular potential

- regulatory mechanisms of hypothalamic-hypophyseal adrenal axis

- regulatory mechanisms of the gas exchange, cardiopulmonary, and detoxification systems

- central nervous system

- autonomic nervous system

Zephyr BioHarness:

The Zephyr BioHarness™ 3 is a physiology-monitoring strap that can be worn in virtually any environment—from combat situations to the sports field. It maintains performance under extreme activity, offering fast, accurate collection and analysis of high-quality, in-depth data. It uses Bluetooth to relay information about the player's physiology to the computer.

Features of the BioHarness include the following:
- long transmission range (about 300 ft up to about 1,000 ft) Bluetooth to provide heart rate, RR interval, speed, and distance to your Android devices

- machine-washable strap that offers both comfort and accuracy

- water resistant up to 1m

- logs and stores up to twenty days of data

- measurements

- HRat

- R-R interval

- breathing rate

- ECG

- posture

- activity level

- peak accel.

Specifications:
- HR range: 25—240 BPM

- BR range: 4–70 BPM

- acc. range: ±16g

- battery type: rechargeable lithium polymer

- battery life: 26 hrs/charge

- charge cycles: 300

References:

(1)   Haldeman, S. Spinal manipulative therapy in sports medicine. *Clin Sports Med* 5(2):277–93, 1986.

(2)   Hoskins, W., and Pollard, H. The effect of a sports chiropractic manual therapy intervention on the prevention of back pain, hamstring and lower limb injuries in semi-elite Australian Rules footballers: a randomized controlled trial. *BMC Musculoskeletal Disorders* 11:64, 2010.

Macquarie Injury Management Group, Department of Chiropractic, Faculty of Science, Macquarie University, NSW 2109, Australia,

(3)   Preliminary investigation of the mechanisms underlying the effects of manipulation: Exploration of a multivariate model including spinal stiffness, multifidus recruitment, and clinical findings. *Spine* 36(21):1772–1781, 1976.

(4)   Fritz, J. M.; Koppenhaver, S. L.; Kawchuk, G. N.; Teyhen, D. S.; Hebert, J. J.; and Childs, J. D.

*Intermountain Healthcare, The University of Utah, Salt Lake City, UT; †US Army-Baylor University Doctoral Program in Physical Therapy (MCCS-HMT), Army Medical Department Center and School, San Antonio, TX; ‡Department of Physical Therapy, University of Alberta, Edmonton, Alberta, CA; §Center for Physical Therapy Research, US Army-Baylor University Doctoral Program in Physical Therapy

(MCCS-HMT), Army Medical Department Center and School, San Antonio, TX; School of Chiropractic and Sports Science, Murdoch University, Murdoch, Western Australia

(5)   Schaefer, J. L.; and Sandrey, M. A. Effects of a 4-week dynamic-balance-training program supplemented with Graston instrument-assisted soft-tissue mobilization for chronic ankle instability. *J Sport Rehabil*. 21(4): 313–326, 2012.

(6)   Looney, B.; Srokose, T.; Fernández-de-las-Peñas, C.; and Graston, J. Instrument soft tissue mobilization and home stretching for the management of plantar heel pain: A case series. *Journal of Manipulative and Physiolog*

(7)   Ramos, G.; and Martin, W. Effects of vertebral axial decompression on intradiscal pressure. *Journal of Neurosurgery*, 81 (3), 350–353, 1994. Retrieved April 19, 2002 from PubMed database.

(8)   Andersson, G. B.; Schults, A. S.; and Nachemson, A. L. Intervertebral disc pressures during traction. *Scand J Rehabil Med* 9:88–91, 1983.

(9)   Gose, E. E.; Naguszewski, W. K.; and Naguszewski, R. K. Vertebral axial decompression therapy for pain associated with herniated or degenerated discs or facet syndrome: An outcome study. *The Journal of Neurological Research*, Volume 20, 1998.

(10)   Tilaro, F.; and Miskovich, D. The effects of vertebral axial decompression on sensory nerve dysfunction in patients with low back pain and radiculopathy. *Canadian Journal of Clinical Medicine* (January 1999).

(11)   Hutchinson, M. *The book of floating: Exploring the private sea.* Nevada City, California: Gateway Books (1984, reprinted 2003).

(12)   Clinical and experimental restricted environmental stimulation: New developments and perspectives (1993), AF Barabasz/M Barabasz, (based on the 4th International Conference on REST), Springer-Verlag New York Inc.

(13)   Restricted environmental stimulation: Research and commentary (1990), TH Fine/JW Turner (based on the 3rd International Conference on REST) Medical College of Ohio Press, Toledo, Ohio.

(14)   Second international conference on REST (1985), TH Fine/JW Turner, IRIS Publications, Toledo, Ohio.

(15)   First international conference on REST and self-regulation (1983), TH Fine/JW Turner, IRIS Publications, Toledo, Ohio.

(16)   Berkoff, D. J.; Cairns, C. B.; Sanchez, L. D.; Moorman, C. T. Heart rate variability in elite American track-and-field athletes. *J Strength Cond Res.* 21(1):227–31, 2007.

Sports Medicine Section, Duke University Medical Center, Durham, North Carolina 27710, USA. david.berkoff@duke.edu

(17)   Mourout 2004.

(18)   Manzi 2009.

The Sixth Pillar

Psychology

The Sixth Pillar: Psychology

SPORTS PSYCHOLOGY REVOLVES AROUND THE PREMISE THAT MENTAL toughness and attitude of the athletes play a major role in the overall outcome of sport, and that it is possible to train the athlete to adopt healthier attitudes through training, repetition, and practice. Sports psychology helps the athlete learn how to identify limiting beliefs, stumbling blocks, and self-doubt and overcome the mental obstacles to success.

The chief aim of psychology in sports is to reduce the level of distraction, improve athletes' confidence, and uplift their overall focus and performance in the game.

Many athletes have an excellent ability to concentrate on certain aspects of sport; that's how they reach the top of the pack. However, in certain scenarios and certain cases, the athlete is either manipulated or restricted by current circumstances and caught up in the drama of life.

In this section of the book, we deal with the tools and techniques that can help the athlete shift focus from undesirable thoughts to desired outcomes.

The main concepts to be dealt with in sports psychology are

1) Self-doubt and self-talk patterns;

2) Anxiety (arousal control);

3) Emotional control;

4) Alcohol/substance abuse; and

5) Focus on desired outcome.

1. Self-doubt:

The performance of athletes depends a great deal on how they think and talk to themselves. Most of the athletes are trained to observe their bodies' behaviors; however, their mental game is either neglected or totally ignored and pushed under the carpet.

The athlete's performance depends a great deal on self-esteem and self-talk. Self-talk has been described by experts as the key to cognitive control. [1]

Self-talk in athletes can be divided into four main types:

- negative ("I'll never get any good at this"; "I'll never be as good as _____")

- positive ("That was great"; "I love my body")

- technical or instructional ("Weight balanced, and breathe!")

- neutral ("What should I eat for dinner?")

Many studies conducted over the last few decades have demonstrated that athletes who have negative self-talk generally display the worst performance, whereas athletes with positive self-talk often display better performance. Elements such as mood, concentration, confidence, and anxiety can be directly influenced by self-talk.

Most of the athletes counseled by sports psychologists suffer from excessive negative self-talk; it is important to note that almost every human being experiences a certain degree of negative self-talk every day; however, when the amount (percentage) of self-talk is high, it can lead to destructive outcomes.

It's estimated that we human beings have an average of sixty thousand thoughts per day; if a mere 10 percent of these thoughts are negative, it could result in six thousand negative thoughts per day! Imagine the plight of an athlete who constantly worries about negative outcomes and experiences 40 percent negative thoughts every day and could be experiencing a total of twenty-four thousand negative thoughts per day.

Now, do you think twenty-four thousand negative thoughts per day could affect the performance of the athletes and sap them of their energy?

Of course it would!

In fact, it could create enough self-doubt that the athlete may forget the initial goal of peak performance and indulge in self-defeating behaviors to avoid facing the reality.

There are many reasons as to why an athlete suffers from negative self-talk:

- trying to think about errors so to fix them, and then dwelling on errors instead of using the lessons learned

- being exposed to a great deal of negative feedback or criticism

- assuming that filtering out positives and perceiving only negatives will help them focus on what needs to be improved

- poor self-image

- expecting perfection in everything and setting unrealistic standards

- engaging in all-or-nothing thinking ("If I can't do this maneuver, then I'm no good") or overgeneralization ("I always lose the important events")

Athletes are constantly told that a positive mental attitude can greatly improve performance; however, it is easier said than done: it takes time, skill, and commitment to change a person's attitude from negative to positive. Many athletes find that the transition from negative to positive is often very difficult and that the concept of self-talk seems unrealistic.

A mix of positive self-talk (self-appreciation and looking for positives) and technical/instructional self-talk (focusing on the task at hand) appears to be the most beneficial method of improving an athlete's mental health.

Using cue words to trigger certain key actions/sports maneuvers during the sports event has also proved useful in competitive situations.

On the other hand, neutral self-talk is often used by endurance athletes to dissociate from the rigors of their event.

The coach must first identify the type of self-talk and the frequency of negative mood before trying to devise a mental-performance plan for the athlete. The following methods can be used to understand the nature of self-talk and its frequency.

Method:

Start an exercise training drill for the athletes that is fairly continuous or repetitive. Explain the process of self-talk and ask the athletes to observe internal thoughts during the drill.

Next ask the athletes to identify every negative thought by raising their hands, to identify every positive thought by clapping their hands twice, and to identify every technical or instructional thought by tapping themselves on the head.

Another method is to use rubber bands for counting thoughts. For example, the athlete may wear two rubber bands—one on each wrist—and may snap the left rubber band whenever a negative thought comes up and snap the right-hand rubber band whenever a positive or technical thought comes up.

You may also point out the fact that such exercises may feel unnatural at first, but it will help the athletes develop a winning attitude over the long term. Ask them to perform the drill to the best of their abilities and to be honest throughout the process.

If you are working one-on-one with an athlete and if you have built enough rapport through prior conversations, you may then proceed to ask the athlete to vocalize each internal thought as it arrives. This is challenging at first, as the athlete may feel self-conscious; however he or she will get used to it.

Record the most significant thoughts that you feel could hinder or improve the athlete's performance.

You may also ask the athletes to record on paper as many of their thoughts as they can at the end of a drill or training session and then classify these thoughts as negative, positive, or technical.

Once the thoughts that need to be worked upon have been identified, then you may use the following drills to reframe the negative thoughts and convert them to something positive that will serve the athlete.

It is beneficial to include such psychological conditioning regimens into your practice and training routine; you may also choose to monitor the improvement and differences in overall performance after two to three weeks of these drills.

Provide enough time for your athletes to practice these exercises, and incorporate them into your training drills whenever possible. After the negative thoughts are identified, they may be reframed using the technique mentioned below.

Common thinking patterns that create negative feelings:

We humans come prewired with a set of standard thinking patterns that create unnecessary mental fog and destroy ambition.

Psychologists call these negative thinking patterns as "cognitive distortions"; below is a list of common cognitive distortions. For a more detailed explanation of cognitive distortions, consider reading *Feeling Good Therapy* by David Burns.

Common cognitive distortions (that create negative emotions):

Style	Description	Example
Filtering	The person identifies and dwells on a single negative detail exclusively.	"I didn't perform well; I missed out on that single shot, and everybody must have noticed it."
All-or-nothing thinking	The person sees things as black or white, with no gray areas in between; the person cannot tolerate anything less than perfect, and sees himself/herself as a total failure.	"I'm very poor with defense positions, which makes me a poor all-rounder, and no team is going to want me."

Overgeneralization	The person sees a single negative event as a never-ending pattern of defeat.	"I always miss important shots."
Jumping to conclusions	Mind-reading: The person jumps to conclusions about people's motives before investigating the truth of the matter. Fortune-telling: The person predicts the worst outcomes and feels convinced that things will turn out badly.	"The spectator looks angry; perhaps he thinks that I'm not playing well." "This travel is going to make me sick."
Magnification and minimization	The person exaggerates the importance of things (such as your error or other's achievements) or minimizing things to appear insignificant (such as your achievements or other's errors).	"I missed the defense on that shot; I'm going to be noted for it, and I will never make it on the final team" or "My performance and physical fitness were good, but I will never be selected because I'm unlucky."
Personalizing	The person perceives everything people do or say as a reaction and always compares himself/herself to others; the person also takes on excessive blame and assumes that he or she is the cause of a negative event that is out of control.	"We lost because of me." "I'll never be successful like him."

Control fallacies	Internal control: I am the cause of the success/ failure. External control: It's out of my hands; it's fate.	"I can make our team win, if they trust in me" or "Don't trust in my ability; we will lose." "The referees are playing favorites, so there can be no way we will win this match."
Copping out	Putting all the blame on others; having a victim mentality	"I would have never taken the risk, but my coach forced me to."
Disqualifying the positive	The person rejects positive experiences by insisting he or she doesn't count for some reason or other.	"Who cares if I can play well; I'm not the coach's favorite."

Reframing exercise:

Negative or destructive thought	Positive or technical adaptation
I always lose the important matches.	I'm a good player; I just need to develop a better strategy to improve my performance in important matches.
I hate these long training routines.	My skill levels are improving every day with these long training routines.

Train the athletes to design self-drills so that they are involved in some form of mental training and practice every day; this will help them learn how to monitor their negative and positive thoughts.

- Ask the athletes to constantly identify desired outcomes instead of dissecting and analyzing the nature of problems.

- Ask the athletes to identify the common situations/themes that trigger negative thoughts, and teach them problem-solving techniques to sort out the situation.

- Help the athletes learn how to improve their confidence levels and self-esteem: many sports psychology books address these issues. Recommended books include Bunker et al. 1993 or Hardy et al. 1998.

- Continuously encourage the athlete to stop overanalyzing situations and practice letting go of negative feelings. Recommended books: *Don't Sweat the Small Stuff* and *Easier Than You Think*, both by Richard Carlson.

Such exercises have a very powerful effect over the long-term change in attitude of the athlete; the trainer must note that any enduring psychological change takes time and effort to achieve, and it is essential to employ psychological techniques constantly to help the athlete get rid of negative thinking patterns.

The language of negativity:

Four "word-patterns" that create negativity in the athlete's mind

Let's have a look at the list of words that cause negativity in athletes. Many of these words are commonly used every day, and yet most of us rarely stop to think about the effect these words have on us.

By choosing the right type of words you gain control over your thoughts and emotions, just as negative words can have a negative impact on our mood, strong positive words can also have an uplifting effect on our mentality and when you have powerful positive thoughts it is very difficult to feel stressed or bad about any situation.

Let's have a look at the list of words that cause stress:

Should:

The word *should* creates unnecessary pressure in many athletes; it creates a ripple effect and causes the athlete to act out of necessity, rather than out of self-expression and confidence. Whenever you use the word *should* in your sentences, you are also making an assumption that the world and your environment "should" operate in a prescribed manner.

Example 1:

I *should* perform well at the upcoming sports event, because I need to win the sponsorship.

Example 2:

I care for my family and their well-being, so they *should* demonstrate the same amount of affection and caring for me.

(If your family doesn't return the same amount of affection, it bothers you.)

Example 3:

I *should* feel motivated to perform better.

However, feeling motivated is similar to charging up your cell-phone battery: the charge will wear out, and you need to recharge again.

Using *should* moves you away from reality; it also burdens your thinking and increases your stress levels.

Instead, replace *should* with *want* and *willing to* in your vocabulary.

You can reframe the above three sentences as follows:

1) I *want* to win the sponsorship at the upcoming sports event, and I am *willing to* work hard for it.

2) I *want* to gain affection from my partner or spouse, and I am *willing to* care for my loved one's well-being.

3) I *want* to exercise consistently for the next six months, and I am *willing to* keep myself motivated.

This reframing allows you to use power words and statements in your language instead of "obligation/expectation" words; such reframing reduces the chances of frustration and keeps you motivated over the long term.

Here are some common situations where we use the word *should*:

o when we talk about our goals in career, health, and relationships

o when we talk about our obligations

o when we talk about our expectations of self and others

o when we impose our belief systems on others

Exercise: Take an inventory of the situations where you are using the words *should* and replace it with the words *want* and *willing to*; notice how the stress levels lower immediately.

Must/have to/has to:

Must, have to and *has to* are pressure words: whenever you use these words, you are trading 90 percent of the control over the situation. If people hear these words, it makes them feel pressurized; it constantly puts people in a stressful do-or-die situation.

Let's look at a few examples:

1) I must start an hour early if I have to make in it time for my training.

2) I <u>must</u> exercise daily to boost my performance.

3) I <u>must</u> make my coach happy or else he won't recommend me.

4) I <u>must</u> take up yoga or meditation to attain mental peace.

5) I <u>have to</u> prepare well in advance for my competition

6) I <u>have to</u> report on time.

7) She <u>has to</u> teach me how to ride the horse.

Do you see how these sentences can increase the stress in your life? Even though all the goals appear worthwhile, the way you frame your goals can have an impact on you mentality.

So then how do you manage and attain your goals without using these pressure words?

Replace the word *must* with the words *prefer to*; the above sentences can then be phrased as follows:

1) I prefer to start an hour early, so that I can make it on time for my training.

2) I prefer to exercise and attain higher performance.

3) I prefer to keep my coach happy, so he considers recommending me.

4) I prefer to take up yoga or meditation, so that I can maintain mental peace.

5) I prefer to prepare well in advance for my competition.

6) I prefer to complete the report on time.

7) I prefer to hire her for learning horse-riding; if it doesn't work out, then I'm willing to consider other options.

The stress-reducing power of vocabulary cannot be underestimated. Thoughts are made up of words, and the words we choose to frame our thoughts can influence the way we feel about different situations.

Cannot:

When you use the word *cannot*, it causes you to focus on the problem instead of the solution; needless to say that this affects your confidence and makes you feel negative.

The secret to true power in life is to know what you *can* do instead of dwelling upon what you *cannot*.

When you dwell upon what you cannot do, you emulate the thinking style of a powerless victim, but when you think about what you *can* do in your circumstance, you will immediately get a grip on reality, and this will help you get rid of unnecessary stress.

Examples:

1) "I cannot keep eating oily and crunchy food all day; it's making me fat."

This can be changed to "I can eat fresh and natural food to maintain my health."

2) "I cannot go away on a vacation, since I'm running out of savings."

This statement can be changed to "I can only take small weekend breaks from work, since I want to maintain my savings."

3) "I cannot work for long hours; it will burn me out."

This can be changed to "I can take small and regular breaks as necessary to avoid burnout."

Take a moment and list out the situations in which you are using the word *cannot* and replace them with the word *can*; this will give you immediate clarity over the situation.

Judgmental words: *Good/Bad, Right/ Wrong:*

When you use judgmental words such as *good/bad* or *right/wrong* to describe people or situations, you immediately join 99 percent of the crowd that labels people and complains about how things don't change.

This kind of pattern restricts your insight and makes your thinking plain and predictable.

Judgmental words such as *good/bad, right/wrong*, and *kind/cunning* can convey a hundred different messages, based on the context and setting.

For example, a court judge being "kind" to a serial murderer may not be admirable, whereas a rich man being "kind" to people who are struggling to make a living may be considered generous and admirable.

The meaning of judgmental words changes according to the context, but the labels we give people are often permanent and misleading.

Our society demands us to use our thinking skills and display different behaviors according to the situation, so it would be unfair to label a person as *good/bad* or kind/cunning.

Instead you can describe a person's behavior along with the context. The sentence "She chooses to ___ in _____ situation" helps you do that.

Example:

"He chooses to be reserved when it comes to hiring coaches."

"She chooses to be casual when it comes to seeking new coaches."

This process may appear very simple on the surface, but, as you practice it, you will learn that it gives you a more accurate view of the situation and makes you curious instead of judgmental.

This method helps you to look into the deeper issues instantly. This creates an environment for meaningful and insightful thinking rather than mechanical judgment.

Such thinking methods reduce our stress and allow us learn faster and communicate better; on the other hand, mechanical thinking forces us to repeat ineffective thinking patterns and narrows our vision!

That brings us to the end of the section on stressful vocabulary; we covered the four main aspects of vocabulary that create stress. Let's do a small exercise now to apply what we've learned. So what I'd like you to do now is take the next fifteen minutes to look at the four main areas of life:

1) Health

2) Wealth (money)

3) Relationships

4) Peace of mind

Go through the above-mentioned areas of life and identify at least one situation in which you are using one or more of the four word patterns, and replace them with the preferred words/sentences; this will instantly nullify any stress you may be experiencing. Carry these statements on a sheet of paper and look at them regularly.

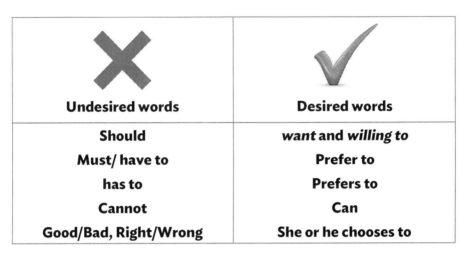

Undesired words	Desired words
Should	*want* and *willing to*
Must/ have to	Prefer to
has to	Prefers to
Cannot	Can
Good/Bad, Right/Wrong	She or he chooses to

If you repeat this exercise daily, you will notice that your attitude becomes completely stress-free and your thinking becomes more clear and flexible.

With practice it will become a regular habit for you to watch and eliminate negative vocabulary from your language. It's important to understand that we interpret the world through our word: the inner dialogue in our minds can either be a good friend or a negative foe, and it's up to us to control our inner dialogue and steer it in a positive direction.

Other psychological techniques:

Autogenic training:
Autogenic training is a form of training that makes your body sensitive to verbal commands. After mastering autogenic training, your body will be able to automatically respond to verbal cues and use them as a switch/trigger for relaxation.

With practice your verbal commands will become powerful enough to control the rate of breathing, heartbeat, blood pressure, and temperature of the body. Since these are the basic elements that control levels of fatigue and alertness, mastering the autogenic technique can prove to be a powerful advantage in the world of competitive sport.

Autogenic training revolves around the premise of six exercises that can make your body warm, relaxed, or heavy. Each exercise is performed while being seated in a standard posture (sitting straight or reclining); it requires you to focus on visually imagining the verbal cues and commanding your body to relax in a certain way.

You may first start by learning about the exercise and then practice it a few times every day to achieve mastery over the concept. Mastering autogenic training can prove to be very beneficial; however, it takes time to master the art of autogenic training; as with other things, autogenic training is a skill that can be developed only through repetition and practice, but the rewards are worth the effort.

Commitment is an essential part of learning autogenic training, because it requires regular practice. Currently autogenic training has been found to be clinically effective in the treatment of the following:

- asthma (including wheezing, coughing and chest tightness)

- hyperventilation (The breathing here is much deeper and rapid than usual; it creates imbalances in oxygenation and leads to feelings of anxiety/stress.)

- bowel movement issues: constipation and diarrhea

- digestion issues: gastritis and stomach spasm

- ulcers

- high blood pressure

- headaches

- cold extremities

- thyroid problems, such as hyperthyroidism

Is autogenic training safe?

Autogenic training (AT) has been found to be safe for most people. Before starting the autogenic training, it might be beneficial to contact your doctor and learn if you suffer from any symptoms that can make autogenic training harmful for you. If you suffer from a serious disease such as diabetes or a heart disease, then it is preferable to use autogenic training only under the supervision of your doctor.

This is important, because blood pressure may change during autogenic training; if you have high or low blood pressure, then it is advisable to have a medical checkup with a nurse or doctor to see if you are benefitting from autogenic training and if your blood pressure is being brought under control.

If you observe that autogenic training provides you certain medical benefits, then please try not to stop any medication you were previously taking; instead consult your doctor and plan on tapering your medication under continuous supervision.

Autogenic training is not recommended for people with severe mental or emotional disorders. You should not feel anxious or restless during the sessions; if you experience such a sensation, then please continue training only under the supervision of a professional AT instructor.

The technique for autogenic training:

(Adapted from the original pioneering work by Schultz, J. H.; Luthe, W.; Ostrander, S.; and Schroeder, L .[1,2,3])

Autogenic training: Basic guidelines

- The results of autogenic training are best if it is practiced in a *quiet* place, alone. The best background music suggested for autogenic training is soft "environmental sounds" such as sounds of the sea/ garden or ethereal New Age background music. Avoid regular forms of music, because the melody, rhythms, and energy of the music can influence the outcome of autogenic training.

- It would be beneficial to wear something loose and to remove your shoes.

- You may also consider lying down flat on your back on a carpeted floor or yoga mat in the initial stages of training. This will improve the perception of heaviness/relaxation in your arms and legs.

  Once you have mastered the autogenic training sequence, you may choose to practice at least one condensed session of your daily autogenic training while sitting (or reclining, with your feet up) in a comfortable chair; you may also choose to do the autogenic training in a position of your choice, which may include sitting, standing, walking, or lying down.

- It is advisable not to eat, drink, or smoke prior to an autogenic training session, because the digestive process begins once you consume food; the blood circulation is diverted to the gut in order to aid the digestion.

- It is important not to stand up too quickly after you finish your practice session; instead, after you finish a session, relax with your eyes closed for a few seconds, and then get up slowly. (You may experience *orthostatic hypotension*—which is a sudden drop in blood pressure due to standing up quickly; it may cause you to feel dizzy or even

	faint.) Instead of standing up immediately, you may try counting backwards from 5 to 1, timed to slow, deep breathing, and then say, "Eyes open. Relaxed and calm. Wide awake." • Some emotions get stored in the body and may manifest with physical symptoms or pain; autogenic training can help you get rid of such ailments; for this reason, during the training, you will be focusing intently on your inner experiences and exclude other external events. Some people do report experiencing a dreamlike, dissociative state during the experience (hypnagogic state); if you experience such a state, do realize that it's completely normal, and let it pass. If are not able to let go of feelings or emotions, then you may consider consulting a psychologist to get rid of any uncomfortable thoughts or feelings.
Training Time	As mentioned earlier, autogenic training takes time and cannot be rushed; therefore, it is important to remember that you may not experience dramatic results during the first few sessions; you may need to repeat certain exercises to achieve the desired results. The chief aim of the training is not to understand the process but instead to feel it and master it. The results are well worth the effort in the long run.
Warm-up routine	## Warm-up routine The warm-up routine prepares your body for the autogenic training; the warm-up routine must be continued even after you master autogenic training. This warm-up involves practicing breathing patterns. Method: For the warm-up you need to start by inhaling for one count and then exhaling for two counts. Try to increase the duration of breathing with each cycle.

	For example, inhale, counting "One"; exhale, counting, "One, two." Inhale, counting, "One, two"; exhale, counting, "One, two, three, four." Go up the scale to six counts in, twelve counts out.
	Then reduce the number of counts per breath in a reverse fashion: six counts in, *twelve counts out;* five counts in, *ten counts out;* and so on, down to one count in, *two counts out.*
Steps of autogenic training: **Step 1: Heaviness**	## Step 1: Heaviness Step 1 of the exercise must be started after the completion of the warm-up phase. Start step 1 with your dominant hand. (If you are right-handed, your dominant hand will be the right hand). Take a deep breath—one count in, one count out—and silently repeat the following formula; the first half of each phrase should be repeated as you inhale (the part before the "/"), the second half should be repeated as you exhale (the part after the "/"): My right arm is getting / limp and heavy 6–8 times My right arm is getting / heavier and heavier 6–8 times My right arm / is completely heavy 6–8 times I feel / completely calm 1 time Repeat this routine two or three times a day, and try to achieve the sensation in your right arm; you may take your time for this process. It is important to note that you will develop control over one limb at a time; therefore, you are advised to train one limb at a time for a period of *three days.* After that, continue with the same basic routine structure, but with another limb, until you achieve control over all your limbs. Here is the suggested routine for training; use the following *substitutions*:

- My *left arm* is getting / limp and heavy, etc. — 3 days

- *Both my arms* are getting / limp and heavy, etc. — 3 days

- My *right leg* is getting / limp and heavy, etc. — 3 days

- My *left leg* is getting / limp and heavy, etc. — 3 days

- *Both my legs* are getting / limp and heavy, etc. — 3 days

- *My arms and legs* are getting / limp and heavy, etc. — 3 days

*The step-1 routine takes twenty-one days
of practice.*

At the end of the twenty-one days, your last cycle of this routine will temporarily be known as your final *heaviness mantra:*

My arms and legs are getting / limp and heavy   6–8 times

My arms and legs are getting / heavier and heavier   6–8 times

My arms and legs are / completely heavy   6–8 times

I feel / completely calm   1 time

Step 2: Warmth

Begin with the *warm-up* breathing exercise. Do the final *heaviness mantra* with all the repetitions. (Heaviness—and the muscular relaxation it represents—is critical to the rest of the training. So you need to master it well right from the start.) At the end of the *heaviness mantra,* add this exercise for warmth:

My right arm is getting / limp and warm   6–8 times

My right arm is getting / warmer and warmer   6–8 times

My right arm / is completely warm   6–8 times

I feel / completely calm   1 time

Practice this routine (the heaviness mantra combined with the warmth exercises) two or three times a day, for *three days.* After that, continue with the same routine structure but with the following substitutions (remembering to do the warm-up breathing exercise and the heaviness mantra at the beginning of each practice session):

- My *left arm* is getting / limp and warm, etc. — 3 days
- *Both my arms* are getting / limp and warm, etc. — 3 days
- My *right leg* is getting / limp and warm, etc. — 3 days
- My *left leg* is getting / limp and warm, etc. — 3 days
- *Both my legs* are getting / limp and warm, etc. — 3 days
- *My arms and legs* are getting / limp and warm, etc. — 3 days

The step-2 routine takes twenty-one days of practice.

At the end of the twenty-one days, you may use a final *heavy/warm mantra* to sum up the first two exercises:

My arms and legs are getting / limp and heavy and warm	6–8 times
My arms and legs are getting / heavier and warmer	6–8 times
My arms and legs are / completely heavy and warm	6–8 times
I feel / completely calm	1 time

Practice this *heavy/warm mantra* (beginning with the warm-up breathing exercise) two or three times a day for one week.

Step 3: A calm heart	## Step 3: A calm heart
	Start with the warm-up. Then begin the following routine, which incorporates your previous work (the heavy/warm mantra) and adds the calm heart exercise:

My arms and legs are getting / limp and heavy and warm	1–2 times
My arms and legs are getting / heavier and warmer	1–2 times
My arms and legs are / completely heavy and warm	1–2 times
I feel / completely calm	1–2 times
My chest feels / warm and pleasant *	6–8 times
My heartbeat is / calm and steady	6–8 times
I feel / supremely calm	6–8 times

* This phrase helps to achieve a calm heart response, but it will be dropped after this exercise.

Practice this routine two or three times a day for two weeks.

Step 4: Breathing	

Step 4: Breathing

Start with the warm-up. Then begin the following routine, which incorporates all your previous work and adds command of your breathing as well:

My arms and legs are getting / limp and heavy and warm	1–2 times
My arms and legs are getting / heavier and warmer	1–2 times
My arms and legs are / completely heavy and warm	1–2 times
My heartbeat is / calm and steady	1–2 times
I feel / completely calm	1–2 times
My breathing is / completely calm	6–8 times
I feel / completely calm	1 time

	Practice this routine two or three times a day for *two weeks*. By this time you will probably have begun to notice some pleasant and surprising effects from your practice. But continue on to further refine your sense of bodily command.
Step 5: Stomach	## Step 5: Stomach Start with the warm-up. Then begin the following routine, which helps you add a radiant feeling of central warmth and peace to your body:

My arms and legs are getting / limp and heavy and warm	1–2 times
My arms and legs are getting / heavier and warmer	1–2 times
My arms and legs are / completely heavy and warm	1–2 times
My heartbeat is / calm and steady	1–2 times
I feel / completely calm	1–2 times
My breathing is / completely calm	1–2 times
I feel / completely calm	1–2 times
My stomach is getting / soft and warm	6–8 times
I feel / completely calm	1 time

Practice this routine two or three times a day for *two weeks*.

Step 6: Cool Forehead	## Step 6: Cool forehead Start with warm-up. Now it's time to move the thinking region (the head) and begin with the following routine, which helps you add a calm, stabilizing sensation of coolness to your forehead:

	My arms and legs are getting / limp and heavy and warm	1–2 times
	My arms and legs are getting / heavier and warmer	1–2 times
	My arms and legs are / completely heavy and warm	1–2 times
	My heartbeat is / calm and steady	1–2 times
	I feel / completely calm	1–2 times
	My breathing is / completely calm	1–2 times
	I feel / completely calm	1–2 times
	My stomach is getting / soft and warm	1–2 times
	I feel / completely calm	1–2 times
	My forehead is / cool	6–8 times
	I feel / completely calm	1 time

Practice this routine two or three times a day for
two weeks.

Completion

Condensed autogenics formula

By this time you will have mastered all the six phases of the basic training. Your final condensed autogenics formula will now be as follows:

Warm-up (as in previous sessions)

My arms and legs are / heavy and warm	1–2 times
My heartbeat and breathing are / calm and steady	1–2 times
My stomach is / soft and warm	1–2 times
My forehead is / cool	1–2 times
I feel / completely calm	1–2 times

Cognitive-affective stress management training:

This form of mental training is very comprehensive and is designed to achieve emotional response control through specific integrated coping responses that involve the cognitive and relaxation responses.

Research studies [4] reveal that this form of training is very beneficial to athletes; they are the ideal candidates for this form of training, because the desired responses such as muscular skills of relaxation are easier to achieve in athletes, who are much more in control of their bodies than are other types of subjects.

These techniques help in anxiety reduction and train the athlete to take into account factors such as actual facts, the mental appraisal of the event, the physiological response generated in the body, and the actual behavior displayed by the subject.

This training has four separate components:

1) Pretreatment assessment: In this phase of training, the consultant will work with the athlete to assess how stress currently affects the athlete's behaviors, and this interview will also assess the player's behavioral skills and shortcomings. This information will help the interviewer prepare a tailor-made program to help the athlete overcome setbacks caused by anxiety and stress.

2) Treatment rationale: During this phase the player receives a detailed explanation of how stress could be affecting the player's performance and how that performance could be improved by the skills learned during this training. It is important to note that this training is more of an educational process and less of a psychotherapy; it is not intended to replace traditional therapy; instead its purpose is to help the athlete

understand the effects of stress on performance and thereby improve the overall output through training.

3) Skill acquisition: The main aim of this training is to help the player develop a complete and comprehensive response mechanism to stress and anxiety; it will teach the subject to modify behavior and look at the existing situation differently.

The diagram below explains the approach taken by this training to help the athlete handle stress better.

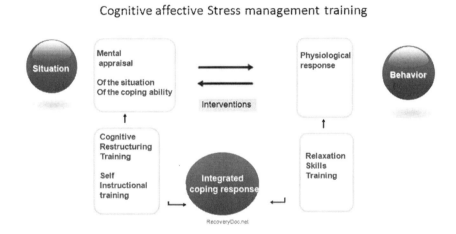

During this phase of training, the athlete will be taught how to achieve muscular relaxation, restructure their thoughts, and will learn the process of self-instruction.

a) Muscular relaxation: This is achieved by training the muscles to relax progressively.

b) Cognitive restructuring: The athlete is taught how to identify irrational/stress-causing self-talk, which may stem from fear of failure or disapproval. The athlete is then taught to restructure these statements into positive thoughts.

The training is also aimed at teaching the athlete useful self commands that can be used in situations that are highly stressful and demanding.

This will help the athlete relax instead of feeling tensed.

4) Skill rehearsal: During this phase of the training process, the consultant will simulate certain stressful situations to test the athlete's coping capabilities and then will help the athlete practice learned skills to cope with the stress.

The consultant may use aids such as films or imaginary rehearsals of stress-inducing situations that may include psychological, emotional, and physiological components that may be found in highly competitive athletic events.

Stress inoculation training (SIT):

Stress inoculation training has proven to produce satisfactory both inside and outside the training zone for athletes. [7] The approach used in stress inoculation training is similar to cognitive affective stress management training. [5, 6]

In SIT the athlete learns how to cope with stress using a ladder pattern of adaptation; that is, the amount of stress experienced by the athlete is gradually increased with each training phase, and the athlete is taught how to cope with increasing levels of stress. After the stressful scenario is simulated, SIT uses a combination of psychological triggers to provoke positive responses; these tools include using productive thoughts, mentally rehearsing positive outcomes, and enhancing well-being with self-statements.

The consultant may also choose to use a four-step approach:

1) Preparation: expecting a stressful situation ahead of time.

2) Expecting real-time emotions and developing positive statements for the moment; for example, "Stay focused, because situations are stacked up against you."

3) Coping with overwhelming feelings; for example, focusing on only the next small step.

4) Evaluation: retrospectively evaluating how you felt and handled the situation. This reinforces self-esteem and boosts the player's confidence; for example, "You handled the situation well."

Throughout this training phase, the athletes develop a capability for learned resourcefulness by learning to cope with events that are increasingly stressful and by completing challenging homework assignments.

How to use arousal-inducing techniques to stimulate performance and recovery in sport:

In the previous section of this book, we talked about various anxiety-reduction techniques; however, anxiety is not the only negative emotion experienced by sport athletes—there is another commonly ignored negative emotion that commonly flies under the radar: the emotion we are talking about is *apathy* or *lack of enthusiasm*.

This lack of enthusiasm may not be a continuous state in athlete; however, it may surface from time to time, causing the athlete to skip a training routine, not take initiative, and eventually give a lackluster performance in sport.

Whenever athletes feel a lack of enthusiasm, they feel lethargic or under-energized.

This may also be seen in situations where the player has taken the opponent too lightly and senses that the opponent does not pose a real threat; it may be seen in situations when the athlete plays a long game and feels mentally exhausted.

The most common approach used by coaches is to give a pep talk and try to boost the morale of the sports athlete; however, this strategy has two flaws: first, it does not have the same effect on all the athletes; second, the coach may exert maximum force in an attempt to motivate all the athletes in the team, and this strategy may lead to excessive arousal, and excessive arousal can make certain players hurried and anxious. The chief aim should be to achieve optimal arousal in such situations; the approach should be deliberate, and the athlete must be self-aware of their arousal states throughout the process.

For this purpose, athletes must first become aware of their low-energy states when they occur and learn how to identify the signs of low energy and low motivation:

1) slow movement around the training/playing circuit

2) easily distracted; signs of mind wandering

3) apathy: unaffected by the quality of performance

4) loss of enthusiasm or eager anticipation

5) feeling heavy in the legs with no bounce in the step

These signs may not be present at all times; however, the frequent presence of these symptoms point to the fact that the athlete is low on arousal and can benefit from arousal-inducing techniques.

When the athlete learns how to track and monitor these signs, the player will develop the ability to detect signs of low energy very early and take appropriate measures to remedy the low energy; continued practice of such techniques can enable the athlete to stay motivated and take on challenging sporting events without getting exhausted or burned out; however, neglecting these signs will push the athlete to burn out much faster and give up much sooner.

Here are some of the most commonly used arousal techniques:

1. ***Increasing breath rate:*** Energy and body tension are directly related to breathing patterns and mental focus; many yoga techniques rely on breathing modifications to achieve states of high awareness and high energy; one of the most commonly used techniques to improve the athlete's energy is an increased rate of breathing. Short, deep breaths are known to activate the nervous system and revitalize the human body.

An increased breathing rate along with short affirmations such as "energy in" with each inhalation and "fatigue out" with each exhalation can produce an energy-elevating effect for athletes.

2. ***Change your physiology:*** Much work and research in the field of neurolinguistic programming has shown that individuals can alter their well-being and state of mind by changing their physiology; pioneering work by leading motivational speakers such as Tony Robbins revolves around the premise that changing the physiology and body posture can significantly alter the mood and the levels of optimism in an individual. Sports psychologists suggest that athletes should look out for instances whenever they feel slow or low on energy and try to encourage themselves to act energized.

Certain specific activities help the athletes to feel energized; in fact, a deeper look at the sporting world reveals that many successful athletes perform these activities unconsciously. These activities include jumping back and forth over a rope to get into an energized state prior to a competition, bumping against the chest pads of another athlete to get into a pumped state, or taking a little jog prior to the event to get the blood pumping—tiny exercises such as these can help athletes turn around their physiological state in a very short period of time. Short bursts of such activities throughout the game can energize athletes and keep the whole team motivated over long stretches of time.

3. *Use vocabulary to aid your arousal:* Research studies have shown that too much thinking can actually be detrimental to peak performance; an analytical or critical review of the game after the performance may help the athlete correct weaknesses, but engaging in perfectionist or overly analytical behaviors during the sport can actually hinder performance; for this reason the athlete is encouraged to use "positive state" words such as *power, strength, energy*, and *activate*. Alternately, the athlete may also choose to use positive statements such as "I'm in peak state," or "My focus is laser-sharp!"

4. *Listen to music:* Recent research studies [8] have proven that many successful athletes use music to stimulate their mood prior to a big game. It's been found that energetic music can have an uplifting effect on the mood of the player, especially if used prior to the game. It is a common practice among players to listen to music on their mp3 players prior to a match.

A recent study [9] found that the amount and type of music preferred by each athlete varies, and that no select genre of music has the same effect on all players; hence the player needs to choose his own music to achieve the desired arousing effect.

5. *Use visualization and imagery:* Imagery is found to be helpful in producing an energized state. The athlete may choose to compare himself

to an efficient object or animal during the competition; for example, a sprinter may imagine a cheetah sprinting effortlessly, and a swimmer may imagine a shark powering its way forward.

6. ***Try a precompetitive workout:*** A precompetitive workout is usually performed four to ten hours prior to a competition and helps the body produce the necessary hormones and chemicals to energize the body; this helps the athlete jump into action on the day of the competition.

Here are some dos and dont's of motivation for sports coaches; these guidelines were created by Lou Holtz, who served as a successful coach for several major colleges:

1) Give players a blueprint for victory; just letting them know that they need to win may not always be well received.

2) Confidence has a major impact on the performance of the team; it is therefore important to give the team the impression that they can win.

3) Players have a knack for lie detection; if players detect that you are lying, then you will lose their respect.

4) Players also have the ability to spot a phony instantly; therefore, it's important to be yourself.

5) Keep the environment lighthearted: it's important to maintain a lighthearted environment and let the team have its share of laughs and jokes; if the players sense a serious do-or-die attitude from the coach, they tend to tighten up very quickly.

Imagery:

Imagery is known to provide the following benefits in athletes:

- Improved concentration: imagery prevents mind-wandering during the sport.

- Enhanced motivation.

- Greater confidence.

- Controlled emotional response.

- Acquisition, practice, and correction of sport skills.

- Better strategy planning.

- Better preparation for competition.

- Better coping with pain and injury.

- Better problem-solving.

Through the use of imagery, an athlete can achieve a state of controlled and relaxed contraction of muscles and modified movements. Imagery helps the athlete maintain positive focus.

Research studies [11] have revealed that positive images of healing or full recovery can enhance the recovery process and speed up recovery times.

Guidelines for using imagery in sport:

Imagery is like any other skill; it can be mastered only through repetitive practice.

Internal vs. external imagery:

Imagery can be of two types: it can be internal or external. In external imagery athletes view themselves as actors in a mental movie; i.e., athletes see themselves performing a desired action; due to this reason, external imagery has a strong visual complement. In internal imagery athletes imagine experiencing the event; therefore, most of the imagery is predominantly kinesthetic.

Research studies [13] on imagery have shown that "visualizing" a biceps curl produces only ocular responses, while "muscularly imagining" the same movement generates localized biceps activity. A significant study on the main effects of imagery revealed that the internal imagery condition produced more integrated biceps activity than the external imagery condition, as predicted by Lang's (1979) bio-informational theory of emotional imagery.

This signifies that external imagery produces very little physiological response when compared to internal imagery; therefore, it may not be effective in enhancing muscular performance.

However, it is important to note that humans regularly switch between internal imagery and external imagery; some athletes may be more kinesthetic, whereas some of them may be visual. While it may be important to illustrate the difference between internal imagery and external imagery and encourage the athletes to adopt internal imagery, the coach must be mindful of the personal preferences of individual athletes and not force them to conform to a particular form of imagery.

The imagery should involve as many sensations as possible: namely sight, sound, smell, touch, and feeling. The athlete should imagine the setting of the sport clearly; this may include the surface of the sporting arena, the surrounding environment, the spectators, etc.

Imagery maybe used during the following times:

- before and after practice

- before and after competition

- during off-season

- during breaks in the action

- during personal time

- when recovering from an injury

Research studies [10] have shown that imagined stimuli and real stimuli have the same effect on the brain and thereby help the brain to learn winning behaviors.

The players must try and imagine the sensations that they are likely to experience during the sporting event; this may include anxiety, excitement, frustration, and exhaustion; the ideal list of emotions would be the emotions that each athlete is familiar with, as this helps the athlete to experience the imagery with more vividness. Having the imagery as close as possible to the real event helps the athlete's brain to accept the imagery and integrate the desired response.

If athletes are unable to imagine the event, they must return to imagining elements of the sport that they are most familiar with and then gradually try and incorporate other details into the imagery. For example, it may be easy for a basketball player to imagine playing on a shiny wooden surface; therefore, the athlete will first spend some time imagining walking and running on the wooden floor; later she or he will introduce more elements one by one.

Consider using the following three preliminary exercises to train the athletes:

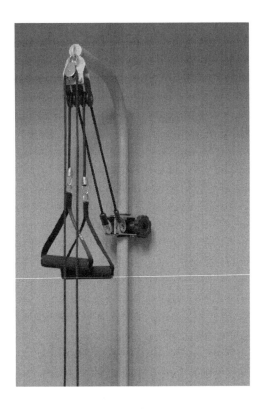

Exercise 1: Ask the athletes to imagine their homes. Ask them to imagine walking into their homes and describing what they see—the color, shape, and texture of things; the sounds, smells, and other sensations related to the room.

Exercise 2: Ask the athletes to imagine performing a skill; they may choose a certain skill that is crucial to the outcome of the sporting event and try to practice the routine perfectly. The athletes should be encouraged to imagine the events as vividly as possible and try to feel the sensations and emotions in their bodies. The players may also try imagining their routines in slow motion and visualize all the details.

Exercise 3: Recall a positive event from the past that is directly related to peak performance. The most important sensations to focus on are the auditory, visual, and kinesthetic aspects of the event.

The athlete may start by imagining the visual aspects of the event, then imagine seeing the opponent, overcoming the challenge, and achieving the positive outcome.

Then the athletes may slowly try and incorporate the auditory signals and imagine the sounds they heard in the sporting arenas, their internal dialogue, and what they were saying to themselves to achieve the winning outcome.

The athletes are then instructed to feel the kinesthetic part of the event; i.e., imagine how they felt physically: the sensations in their bodies and the excitement, anxiety, or challenge.

Sport-specific guidelines:

Volleyball: Use imagery before matches.

Method: Reserve a quiet, dark room where players can visualize themselves performing against a specific opponent.

Basketball: Use imagery before practice.

Method: Have players imagine their specific assignments for different defenses and offensive sets.

Tennis: Use imagery during changeovers.

Method: Instruct players to visualize what type of strategy and shots they want to use in the upcoming game.

Swimming: Use imagery after every practice.

Method: Give swimmers five minutes to pick a certain stroke, and ask them to imagine doing it perfectly, or have them visualize it during rest periods between intervals.

Dealing with mental exhaustion: Overtraining and burnout in sport:

Overtraining can be defined as a short cycle of training during which athletes expose themselves to excessive training loads that are near to or at maximal capacity.

Most of the sporting world is driven by adrenaline; oftentimes the pressure to exhibit extraordinary performance in sport pushes the player to take the training too far; the athlete often struggles to keep up the quest for being the ultimate champion, and this quest (even though it is positive and worthwhile) can push the athlete to overtraining.

Overtraining can lead to either staleness or burnout.

Staleness can be defined as a physiological state of overtraining that manifests as deteriorated athletic readiness (AMA 1966). The stale athlete has a 5 percent reduction in performance that persists for two weeks or longer.

Burnout is an exhaustive psychophysiological response exhibited as a result of frequent, sometimes extreme, and generally ineffective efforts to meet excessive training and competitive demands.

These conditions usually result from many different factors, which include high levels of fatigue, poor immune system, high levels of emotional or physical stress, and poor knowledge about recovery.

Burnout can lead to a variety of undesirable effects:

- low levels of enthusiasm or ambition
- trouble with completing usual routines
- changes in sleep patterns (more or less sleep than usual)

- decreased appetite and/or weight loss

- increased injuries, illness, or infections

- decreased sports and/or school performance

- chronic muscle or joint pain

- changes in personality or mood

- elevated resting heart rate

- constant fatigue

Quick tips to avoid burnout:

Use the following strategies and tips to reduce the chances of burnout:

Plan long-term: The entire training schedule of the athlete can be divided into three to four training phases that are spread throughout the year. The athlete may then be given quarterly goals to achieve; the progress may be monitored on a weekly basis.

Promote cross-training: Encourage athletes to vary their workouts throughout the training regimen; athletes may focus on different aspects such as conditioning, weight lifting, strength training, flexibility, or core strengthening at different times during their training phase.

Technique correction: Encourage the athlete to use the correct technique for training at all times; this will ensure that the damage from wear and tear during sport is minimal.

Focus on slow gain: Even though rapid progress may appear to be attractive, the effects may be temporary, and the athlete may face undue levels of stress; instead a slow progression with a gradual increase in workload or intensity will improve the capacity of the athlete and promote endurance.

Adopt a continuous holistic education schedule and inform the athletes about the best tools, mind-sets, and techniques to enjoy high levels of sportsmanship, safety, fitness, and all-round performance. Such a continuous education program will prevent the athlete from becoming one-dimensional.

Emphasize proper injury treatment and rehabilitation:

- High stress in life is associated with higher injury rates in sports due to several factors such as attention disruption (reduced attention span), increased muscle tension (muscle tension interferes with normal coordination and biomechanics and thus increases chance for injury), and poor care.

- It is therefore important to educate the injured person about the injury and recovery process. The injured athlete may benefit from psychological coping skills (goal-setting, positive self-talk, imagery visualization, and relaxation training) and a better rapport with the coach.

References:

(1)   Schultz, J. H.; and Luthe, W. *Autogenic training: A psychophysiologic approach in psychotherapy*. New York: Grune and Stratton. 1959.

(2)   Schultz, J. H.; and Luthe, W. *Autogenic therapy: Vol. 1. Autogenic methods*. New York: Grune and Stratton. 1969.

(3) The autogenics exercises presented here have been adapted from Ostrander, S., and Schroeder, L. *Superlearning*. New York: Dell Publishing Co. 1979.

(4) Crocker, Alderman, Murray and Smith 1988

(5) Kerr and Leith 1993

(6) Kerr and Goss 1996

(7) Meichenbaum 1985

(8) Bishop, Karageorghis, and Loizou 2007

(9) Mann, Edmonds, Tenenbaum, and Janelle 2006

(10) Marks 1977, p 285

(11) Levleva and Orlick 1991

(12) The effects of internal and external imagery on muscular and ocular concomitants. *JSEP Sport Psychology* 4(4): 379–387.

(13) Mahoney and Avener's (1977) categorization of imagery

Conclusion:

I hope you enjoyed the book and learned new insights from it.

You don't have to go on this journey alone; I'll be writing to you regularly through our newsletter and blog, and we also have many programs and training sessions for those who want to learn new skills and stay at the cutting edge of sports medicine.

As an owner of this guide, you will also be receiving firsthand updates and special tips from me that no one else will get.

I'd like it very much if you'd stay in touch with me. Share your comments and personal experience; ask me for suggestions, advice, or professional assistance.

Visit my website regularly, and contact me any time at my personal email: rrosadc@gmail.com.

Implement what you have learned in this book; contact me in ninety days, then again in six months, and again in a year to tell me how you're doing! I want to hear your success story, and I'd love to get a testimonial; you have the opportunity to inspire other athletes and trainers with your results.

I congratulate you and salute you on your conquests, and I look forward to a long-lasting friendship.

Your friend,

Rick Rosa

www.recoverydoc.net

rrosadc@gmail.com

Blog http://www.recoverydoctor.blogspot.com/

Twitter @drrickrosa

Made in the USA
San Bernardino, CA
28 September 2013